Mark S. Gold, MD
Editor

Smoking
and Illicit Drug Use

Smoking and Illicit Drug Use has been co-published simultaneously as *Journal of Addictive Diseases*, Volume 17, Number 1 1998.

Pre-publication
REVIEWS,
COMMENTARIES,
EVALUATIONS . . .

"**N**ot only links cigarette use to alcohol and illicit drug use, but points the way for society to harness the fear of addiction to help both prevent and treat nicotine addiction. Based on an understanding of the brain biology of reward, Gold and his colleagues provide policymakers, clinicians, and the public with the best ever look at the reason why 90% of the nation's more than 60 million cigarette smokers want to quit but have trouble achieving that life-saving goal."

Robert L. DuPont, MD
President
Institute for Behavior and Health
Professor of Psychiatry
Georgetown University School of Medicine
Rockville, MD

Smoking
and Illicit Drug Use

Smoking and Illicit Drug Use has been co-published simultaneously as *Journal of Addictive Diseases*, Volume 17, Number 1 1998.

Alcohol Research from Bench to Bedside, edited by Enoch Gordis, Boris Tabakoff, and Markku Linnoila*

Addiction Potential of Abused Drugs and Drug Classes, edited by Carlton K. Erikson, Martin A. Javors, and William W. Morgan*

Behavioral and Biochemical Issues in Substance Abuse, edited by Frank R. George and Doris Clouet*

Cocaine, AIDS, and Intravenous Drug Use, edited by Samuel R. Friedman and Douglas S. Lipton

What Works in Drug Abuse Epidemiology, edited by Blanche Frank and Ronald Simeone

Cocaine: Physiological and Physiopathological Effects, edited by Alfonso Paredes and David A. Gorlick

Comorbidity of Addictive and Psychiatric Disorders, edited by Norman S. Miller

Experimental Therapeutics in Addiction Medicine, edited by Stephen Magura and Andrew Rosenblum

The Effectiveness of Social Interventions for Homeless Substance Abusers, edited by Gerald J. Stahler and Barry Stimmel

The Neurobiology of Cocaine Addiction: From Bench to Bedside, edited by Herman Joseph and Barry Stimmel

Intensive Outpatient Treatment for the Addictions, edited by Edward Gottheil

The Integration of Pharmacological and Nonpharmacological Treatments in Drug/Alcohol Addictions, edited by Norman S. Miller

Smoking and Illicit Drug Use, edited by Mark S. Gold

These books were published simultaneously as special thematic issues of the *Journal of Addictive Diseases* and are available bound separately. Visit Haworth's website at http://www.haworth.com to search our online catalog for complete tables of contents and ordering information for these and other publications. Or call 1-800-HAWORTH (outside US/Canada: 607-722-5857), Fax: 1-800-895-0582 (outside US/Canada: 607-771-0012) or e-mail getinfo@haworth.com

Smoking
and Illicit Drug Use

Mark S. Gold, MD
Editor

Barry Stimmel, MD
Series Editor

Smoking and Illict Drug Use has been co-published simultaneously as *Journal of Addictive Diseases*, Volume 17, Number 1 1998.

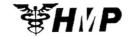

The Haworth Medical Press
An Imprint of
The Haworth Press, Inc.
New York • London

Published by

The Haworth Medical Press, 10 Alice Street, Binghamton, NY 13904-1580 USA

The Haworth Medical Press is an imprint of The Haworth Press, Inc., 10 Alice Street, Binghamton, NY 13904-1580 USA.

Smoking and Illicit Drug Use has been co-published simultaneously as *Journal of Addictive Diseases*, Volume 17, Number 1 1998.

The development, preparation, and publication of this work has been undertaken with great care. However, the publisher, employees, editors, and agents of The Haworth Press and all imprints of The Haworth Press, Inc., including The Haworth Medical Press and The Pharmaceutical Products Press, are not responsible for any errors contained herein or for consequences that may ensue from use of materials or information contained in this work. Opinions expressed by the author(s) are not necessarily those of The Haworth Press, Inc.

Cover design by Thomas J. Mayshock Jr.

Library of Congress Cataloging-in-Publication Data

Smoking and illicit drug use / Mark S. Gold, editor.
      p. cm.
      "Co-published simultaneously as Journal of addictive diseases, vol. 17, no. 1, 1998.
      Includes bibliographical references and index.
      ISBN 0-7890-0507-7 (alk. paper)
      1. Tobacco habit. 2. Substance abuse. I. Gold, Mark S. II. Journal of addictive diseases.
RC567.S634 1998
516.86'5–DC21
                                                      97-52072
                                                     CIP

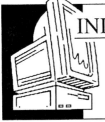

INDEXING & ABSTRACTING

Contributions to this publication are selectively indexed or abstracted in print, electronic, online, or CD-ROM version(s) of the reference tools and information services listed below. This list is current as of the copyright date of this publication. See the end of this section for additional notes.

- *Abstracts in Anthropology,* Baywood Publishing Company, 26 Austin Avenue, P.O. Box 337, Amityville, NY 11701

- *Abstracts of Research in Pastoral Care & Counseling,* Loyola College, 7135 Minstrel Way, Suite 101, Columbia, MD 21045

- *Academic Abstracts/CD-ROM,* EBSCO Publishing Editorial Department, P.O. Box 590, Ipswich, MA 01938-0590

- *ADDICTION ABSTRACTS,* National Addiction Centre, 4 Windsor Walk, London SE5 8AF, England

- *ALCONLINE Database,* Centralforbundet for Alcohol-och narkotikaupplysning, Box 70412, 107 25 Stockholm, Sweden

- *Behavioral Medicine Abstracts,* University of Washington, Department of Social Work & Speech & Hearing Sciences, Box 354900, Seattle, WA 98195

- *Biosciences Information Service of Biological Abstracts (BIOSIS),* Biosciences Information Service, 2100 Arch Street, Philadelphia, PA 19103-1399

- *Brown University Digest of Addiction Theory and Application, The (DATA Newsletter),* Project Cork Institute, Dartmouth Medical School, 14 South Main Street, Suite 2F, Hanover, NH 03755-2015

- *Cambridge Scientific Abstracts,* Health & Safety Science Abstracts, 7200 Wisconsin Avenue #601, Bethesda, MD 20814

- *Child Development Abstracts & Bibliography,* University of Kansas, 213 Bailey Hall, Lawrence, KS 66045

- *CNPIEC Reference Guide: Chinese National Directory of Foreign Periodicals,* P.O. Box 88, Beijing, Peoples Republic of China

- *Criminal Justice Abstracts,* Willow Tree Press, 15 Washington Street, 4th Floor, Newark, NJ 07102

- *Criminal Justice Periodical Index,* University Microfilms, Inc., P.O. Box 32770, Louisville, KY 40232

(continued)

- *Criminology, Penology and Police Science Abstracts,* Kugler Publications, P.O. Box 11188, 1001 GD Amsterdam, The Netherlands

- *Current Contents . . . .* see: *Institute for Scientific Information*

- *Educational Administration Abstracts (EAA),* Sage Publications, Inc., 2455 Teller Road, Newbury Park, CA 91320

- *Excerpta Medica/Secondary Publishing Division,* Elsevier Science Inc., Secondary Publishing Division, 655 Avenue of the Americas, New York, NY 10010

- *Family Studies Database (online and CD/ROM),* National Information Services Corporation, 306 East Baltimore Pike, 2nd Floor, Media, PA 19063

- *Health Source: Indexing & Abstracting of 160 selected health related journals, updated monthly,* EBSCO Publishing, 83 Pine Street, Peabody, MA 01960

- *Health Source Plus: expanded version of "Health Source" to be released shortly:* EBSCO Publishing, 83 Pine Street, Peabody, MA 01960

- *Index Medicus,* National Library of Medicine, 8600 Rockville Pike, Bethesda, MD 20894

- *Index to Periodical Articles Related to Law,* University of Texas, 727 East 26th Street, Austin, TX 78705

- *Institute for Scientific Information,* 3501 Market Street, Philadelphia, PA 19104-3302. Coverage in:
    a) Social Science Citation Index (SSCI): print, online, CD-ROM
    b) Research Alerts (current awareness service)
    c) Social SciSearch (magnetic tape)
    d) Current Contents/Social & Behavioral Sciences (weekly current awareness service)

- *International Pharmaceutical Abstracts,* ASHP, 7272 Wisconsin Avenue, Bethesda, MD 20814

- *INTERNET ACCESS (& additional networks) Bulletin Board for Libraries ("BUBL"), coverage of information resources on INTERNET, JANET, and other networks.*
    - <URL:http://bubl.ac.uk/>
    - The new locations will be found under <URL:http://bubl.ac.uk/link/>.
    - Any existing BUBL users who have problems finding information on the new service should contact the BUBL help line by sending e-mail to <bubl@bubl.ac.uk>.
    The Andersonian Library, Curran Building, 101 St. James Road, Glasgow G4 0NS, Scotland

- *Medication Use STudies (MUST) Database,* The University of Mississippi, School of Pharmacy, University, MS 38677

(continued)

- *Mental Health Abstracts (online through DIALOG),* IFI/Plenum Data Company, 3202 Kirkwood Highway, Wilmington, DE 19808

- *NIAAA Alcohol and Alcohol Problems Science Database (ETOH),* National Institute on Alcohol Abuse and Alcoholism, 1400 Eye Street NW, Suite 600, Washington, DC 20005

- *PASCAL, c/o Institute de L'Information Scientifique et Technique,* Cross-disciplinary electronic database covering the fields of science, technology & medicine. Also available on CD-ROM, and can generate customized retrospective searches. For more information: INIST, Customer Desk, 2, allee du Parc de Brabois, F-54514 Vandoeuvre Cedex, France; http//www.inist.fr

- *Psychological Abstracts (PsycINFO),* American Psychological Association, P.O. Box 91600, Washington, DC 20090-1600

- *Sage Family Studies Abstracts (SFSA),* Sage Publications, Inc., 2455 Teller Road, Newbury Park, CA 91320

- *Sage Urban Studies Abstracts (SUSA),* Sage Publications, Inc., 2455 Teller Road, Newbury Park, CA 91320

- *Social Planning/Policy & Development Abstracts (SOPODA),* Sociological Abstracts, Inc., P.O. Box 22206, San Diego, CA 92192-0206

- *Social Work Abstracts,* National Association of Social Workers, 750 First Street NW, 8th Floor, Washington, DC 20002

- *Sociological Abstracts (SA),* Sociological Abstracts, Inc., P.O. Box 22206, San Diego, CA 92192-0206

- *SOMED (social medicine) Database,* Landes Institut fur Den Offentlichen Gesundheitsdienst NRW, Postfach 20 10 12, D-33548 Bielefeld, Germany

- *Studies on Women Abstracts,* Carfax Publishing Company, P.O. Box 25, Abingdon, Oxon, OX14 3UE, United Kingdom

- *Violence and Abuse Abstracts: A Review of Current Literature on Interpersonal Violence (VAA),* Sage Publications, Inc., 2455 Teller Road, Newbury Park, CA 91320

(continued)

SPECIAL BIBLIOGRAPHIC NOTES

related to special journal issues (separates)
and indexing/abstracting

☐ indexing/abstracting services in this list will also cover material in any "separate" that is co-published simultaneously with Haworth's special thematic journal issue or DocuSerial. Indexing/abstracting usually covers material at the article/chapter level.

☐ monographic co-editions are intended for either non-subscribers or libraries which intend to purchase a second copy for their circulating collections.

☐ monographic co-editions are reported to all jobbers/wholesalers/approval plans. The source journal is listed as the "series" to assist the prevention of duplicate purchasing in the same manner utilized for books-in-series.

☐ to facilitate user/access services all indexing/abstracting services are encouraged to utilize the co-indexing entry note indicated at the bottom of the first page of each article/chapter/contribution.

☐ this is intended to assist a library user of any reference tool (whether print, electronic, online, or CD-ROM) to locate the monographic version if the library has purchased this version but not a subscription to the source journal.

☐ individual articles/chapters in any Haworth publication are also available through the Haworth Document Delivery Service (HDDS).

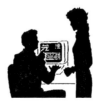

Smoking and Illicit Drug Use

CONTENTS

ALL HAWORTH MEDICAL PRESS BOOKS
AND JOURNALS ARE PRINTED
ON CERTIFIED ACID-FREE PAPER

ABOUT THE EDITOR

Mark S. Gold, MD, is Professor at the University of Florida College of Medicine's Brain Institute, Departments of Neuroscience, Psychiatry, Community Health, and Family Medicine. He is a Fellow of the American College of Clinical Pharmacology (FCP) and of the American Psychiatric Association (FAPA). He is a regular member of the College on Problems of Drug Dependence and a Diplomat of the American Board of Forensic Medicine. Dr. Gold has worked closely with the DEA, has been an active Consultant to the Attorney General's Office, and has been active in drug education and prevention. He has had an active role in the development of core competencies for addiction medicine and the development of standardized cases used throughout the United States to train health professionals. Dr. Gold has authored over 700 medical articles, chapters, and abstracts and is the author of several books, including *800-Cocaine* and *The Good News About Depression*.

EDITORIAL

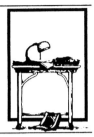

Smoking and Illicit Drug Use–
A Lesson Yet to Be Learned

It may appear to belabor the obvious to observe that nicotine is an addictive substance. Indeed, almost a decade ago, similarities in nicotine dependence to those of heroin and cocaine were published by the Surgeon General.[1] Nonetheless, despite this knowledge, cigarette smoking has continued and, in some instances, has flourished. In adults this initially was not the case, with the average consumption of cigarettes declining dramatically between 1981 and 1993.[2] However, between 1993 and 1994, this decrease plateaued and, since then, cigarette consumption has actually increased, specifically among teenagers. Current smoking among students in grades 9-12 has increased from 27% in 1991 to 34.8% in 1995. This

[Haworth co-indexing entry note]: "Smoking and Illicit Drug Use–A Lesson Yet to Be Learned." Stimmel, Barry, and Mark S. Gold. Co-published simultaneously in *Journal of Addictive Diseases* (The Haworth Medical Press, an imprint of The Haworth Press, Inc.) Vol. 17, No. 1, 1998, pp. 1-5; and: *Smoking and Illicit Drug Use* (ed: Mark S. Gold, and Barry Stimmel) The Haworth Medical Press, an imprint of The Haworth Press, Inc., 1998, pp. 1-5. Single or multiple copies of this article are available for a fee from The Haworth Document Delivery Service [1-800-342-9678, 9:00 a.m. - 5:00 p.m. (EST). E-mail address: getinfo@haworth.com].

observation is exceptionally important as 90% of all persons who initiate the use of tobacco do so under 18 years of age.[3]

Considering the age at which smoking is usually initiated, it is also less than surprising that tobacco, along with alcohol, are the most common "gateway" drugs to use of illicit mood-altering substances. The figure of 400,000 deaths due to smoking has been extensively publicized; however, less well realized, though nonetheless true, is that the number of deaths attributable to smoking in this country is more than 60-fold that seen due to heroin and cocaine use combined. It is therefore less than understandable that only recently have those committed to treating the more commonly recognized addictions, such as alcohol, heroin, and cocaine, become somewhat active in addressing the often coexisting nicotine dependency. This disinterest at times has even facilitated cigarette smoking and nicotine addiction by allowing smoking in inpatient facilities, ostensibly to relieve the anxiety of withdrawal from other drugs.

Fortunately, the addictive properties of the numerous constituents of tobacco smoke and nicotine can now no longer be dismissed due to the recently released information, long held by tobacco companies, demonstrating the addictive qualities of this drug. What is now needed, however, is the accumulation of knowledge by those dealing with addictive behaviors as to the biological mechanisms of nicotine dependence, the prevalence of this dependency among those using other mood-altering drugs, and the most efficacious way to address this dependency. It is therefore quite appropriate that this collection focuses on these aspects of nicotine dependency and on the inhalation of tobacco smoke.

The biologic basis for dependence to nicotine is reviewed by Gold and Herkov, who demonstrate how dependence to this substance is little different from that seen with heroin and cocaine, involving stimulation of the neurotransmitter dopamine in the reward system of the brain.[4] The effects that this has on behavior, as well as the biological explanation of nicotine withdrawal, are also reviewed. This is followed by the rationale for use of pharmacologic therapy for nicotine dependence. The paper by Fowler and colleagues focuses on the specific action of nicotine on monoamine oxidase B in brain tissue, utilizing image analysis with PET scans.[5] These investigators have demonstrated that the inhibition of this enzyme may be responsible for the activation of the brain dopamine system and, ironically, may also be responsible for the observation concerning the ability of nicotine to slow the progression of Parkinson's disease with L-deprenyl. The use of substances that inhibit the subtype of monoamine oxidase (MAO) A inhibitors may actually facilitate smoking cessation in those who are highly dependent on nicotine.

A better understanding of the neurobiological basis of cigarette smoking leads to the question of its relevance to other addictive behaviors. Is the prevalence of smoking greater among those dependent on other mood-altering substances, or is it merely a general sign of anxiety and depression that defines a variety of psychologic dysfunctions? Covey et al. review the literature demonstrating an association between cigarette smoking and major depression and the vulnerability of those with major depression to continue smoking even after achieving abstinence, suggesting that smoking cessation programs must focus on those most at risk for relapse once abstinence has been achieved.[6] Hays et al., in a small but interesting paper, show that, although smoking is increased among those with psychologic problems, in fact both the quantity of caffeine consumed and of cigarettes smoked is indeed increased in those with drug dependence as compared to those with specific psychiatric disorders but no drug dependence.[7] Emphasizing that dependence to nicotine is of special importance in those using other mood-altering drugs, Miller and Gold confirm the association of simultaneous use of cigarettes and other drugs, describing the expected interactions between these substances to increase mortality and morbidity.[8] Their observations of the high rates of mortality from tobacco found in former alcoholics should dispel the thought that tobacco use is only of concern in those currently addicted to alcohol or other mood altering substances.

The paper by Manwell and colleagues describes the prevalence of tobacco, alcohol, and drug use in a general population treated by primary care clinicians.[9] This is quite important as it is the primary care physician who has the opportunity to identify the potential for the existence of nicotine dependency and to take specific action through primary and secondary prevention efforts. Yet surveys have shown that only 25% of teenagers seeing a physician said that information was provided concerning cigarette smoking,[10] with only 50% of smokers reporting that this habit was discussed by their physicians.[11] In a survey of over 21,000 adults, they noted that the prevalence of tobacco use was 27%, with 20% at risk for alcohol-related problems and 5% currently using illicit drugs. Despite the fact that 80% of those who were smokers realized smoking was a problem, and 88% felt that they should diminish their habit, 71% still would awaken in the morning craving a cigarette. The observations gleaned from these papers demonstrate that smoking not only is a problem among the general population but, indeed, is accentuated in those dependent on other drugs.

With this in mind, the paper by Rustin, describing how an addiction treatment program was developed to address nicotine dependence as another drug dependency, is particularly helpful.[12] The author demonstrates not only how an inpatient addiction facility can become smoke-free but, equally important, how continued commitment is needed to maintain this environment. Although the proportion of persons completing treatment declined considerably following the transition to a smoke-free environment, within three months the program completion rate had returned to its usual level for both smokers and nonsmokers, and, after seventeen months in a smoke-free environment, the completion rate was higher than that seen in the past, increasing from 49% to 62% (P < 0.01), with no difference being detected between smokers and nonsmokers. These data serve to correct the often quoted misconception that to abstain from nicotine at a time when abstinence is trying to be achieved from other mood-altering substances will result in a failed therapeutic effort.

Taken together, the papers in this collection describe the biological basis of cigarette smoking as well as how this knowledge can be used to develop approaches to treatment. Smoking produces acute and chronic changes in critical brain systems. Smoking cessation is more complex and difficult than previously thought. Just as no one would propose benzodiazepines or clonidine as treatments for alcoholism or other addictions, the use of pure nicotine is not a treatment but a process to assist in detoxification. We need to get beyond detoxification to improve success. The prevalence of smoking among those engaged in other addictive behaviors is clearly demonstrated, as is a successful model for addressing this issue in a drug treatment facility. Smokers have been seen as merely having a bad habit. This point of view has conspired to confirm the smokers' state of denial and must be addressed. It is ironic that those of us engaged in treatment of the addictions have long ignored the therapeutic means of addressing a dependency to a drug no less intense than heroin or cocaine, yet responsible for more morbidity and mortality than all illicit substances combined.

Barry Stimmel, MD
Mark S. Gold, MD

REFERENCES

1. U.S. Department of Health and Human Services Office of Smoking and Health. The health consequences of smoking: nicotine addiction. A report of the Surgeon General. Washington, DC: U.S. Government Printing Office 1988; 270: 334-335.

2. Cigarette Smoking Among Adults–United States 1994. JAMA. 1996; 276:595-596.

3. Tobacco use and usual source of cigarettes among high school students–United States 1995. Morbidity and Mortality Weekly Report, May 24, 1996; 45(20):413.

4. Gold MS, Herkov MJ. Tobacco smoking and nicotine dependence: biological basis for pharmacotherapy from nicotine to treatments that prevent relapse. J Addict Dis. 1998; 17(1):7-21.

5. Fowler JS, Volkow ND, Wang G-J, Pappas N, Logan J, MacGregor R, Alexoff D, Wolf AP, Warner D, Cilento R, Zezulkova I. Neuropharmacological actions of cigarette smoke: brain monoamine oxidase B (MAO B) inhibition. J Addict Dis. 1998; 17(1):23-34.

6. Covey LS, Glassman AH, Stetner F. Cigarette smoking and major depression. J Addict Dis. 1998; 17(1):35-46.

7. Hays LR, Farabee D, Miller W. Caffeine and nicotine use in an addicted population. J Addict Dis. 1998; 17(1):47-54.

8. Miller NS, Gold MS. Comorbid cigarette and alcohol addiction: epidemiology and treatment. J Addict Dis. 1998;17(1):55-66.

9. Manwell LB, Fleming MF, Johnson K, Barry KL. Tobacco, alcohol, and drug use in a primary care sample: 90-day prevalence and associated factors. J Addict Dis. 1998; 17(1):67-81.

10. Health care provider advice on tobacco use to persons aged 10-22 years. United States 1993. Morbidity and Mortality Weekly Report, November 10, 1995;44:826-830.

11. Heam W. Why don't smokers quit? Am Med News, December 27,1993, pp 7-8.

12. Rustin TA. Incorporating nicotine dependence into addiction treatment. J Addict Dis. 1998; 17(1):83-108.

Tobacco Smoking and Nicotine Dependence: Biological Basis for Pharmacotherapy from Nicotine to Treatments that Prevent Relapse

Mark S. Gold, MD
Michael J. Herkov, PhD, ABPP

INTRODUCTION

Smoking cigarettes is directly linked to over 400,000 deaths in the U.S. each year due to cancer, stroke and cardiovascular disease. Yet cigarettes are only the delivery system for the drug nicotine much as the hypodermic needle and glass bottle provide the heroine addict or alcoholic with their respective drugs. Studies have conclusively shown that smoking tobacco, like smoking heroin or cocaine is profoundly addictive. The neural pathways of the brain's reward system are the same for tobacco as for other drugs, making research from these studies applicable to understanding nicotine addiction. In this paper we will discuss what the DSM-IV de-

Mark S. Gold is Professor, Departments of Neuroscience, Psychiatry, Community Health and Family Medicine, University of Florida Brain Institute, Gainesville, FL.

Michael J. Herkov is Associate Professor, Department of Psychiatry, University of Florida, Gainesville, FL.

[Haworth co-indexing entry note]: "Tobacco Smoking and Nicotine Dependence: Biological Basis for Pharmacotherapy from Nicotine to Treatments that Prevent Relapse." Gold, Mark S., and Michael J. Herkov. Co-published simultaneously in *Journal of Addictive Diseases* (The Haworth Medical Press, an imprint of The Haworth Press, Inc.) Vol. 17, No. 1, 1998, pp. 7-21; and: *Smoking and Illicit Drug Use* (ed: Mark S. Gold, and Barry Stimmel) The Haworth Medical Press, an imprint of The Haworth Press, Inc., 1998, pp. 7-21. Single or multiple copies of this article are available for a fee from The Haworth Document Delivery Service [1-800-342-9678, 9:00 a.m. - 5:00 p.m. (EST). E-mail address: getinfo@haworth.com].

scribes as nicotine dependence and withdrawal from both the psychosocial and neurobiological perspective. Using this knowledge we will review current treatments as well as recommendations for relapse prevention.

NICOTINE ADDICTION/DEPENDENCE

Substance addiction is understood as a preoccupation with the drug, pathological attachment to the drug and brain reinforcement or reward from the drug. Central to this definition is the idea of relapse, or the person's return to the drug after periods of abstinence or significantly curtailed use. Rather than being seen as a moral weakness, recent research has shown that neurobiological changes in the brain associated with drug use set the stage for relapse. Drug use creates a new level of brain reward or pleasure that becomes defined as normal and any attempt to reduce this stimulation through substance abstinence leads to a decreased level of pleasure or anhedonia. Use, therefore, continues as an automatic behavior, even in the absence of consciously reported drug-induced euphoria. It seems as though the addict now uses the drug not for the "high" per se, but as a means to remain what they describe as "normal." Thus, normal becomes defined as presence of the drug and it "abnormal" for the user to abstain from the drug once neuroadaptive changes have occurred. Addiction then is a brain disease where drugs of abuse cause changes to occur in the brain which make additional use more likely to occur. Relapse may be automatic, unconscious and just seem normal at the time.

Nicotine addiction is a complex process involving the interplay of pharmacology, pre-existing hard-wired brain systems for reward, learned or conditioned factors, personality and social settings.[1] Each factor is important in the development of addiction; yet, it is the actual neurobiological process of addiction which locks a person into a pattern of addiction. The biological process is the least understood among those listed and it is perhaps the most important given our lack of success curing addiction. Our improving understanding of the mechanisms of addiction has already yielded promising pharmacologic treatments targeted specifically at the rewarding aspects of addiction.[2]

We know that the pattern of tobacco addiction typically begins in teenage years. Young people begin smoking for various psycho-social reasons: peer pressure, easy access, parental role models, defiance, and image of maturity. Repeated use leads to some tolerance and desensitizes the smoker to some of the aversive effects of smoking, including nausea. Studies of nicotinic receptors in the brain have been correlated with this effect.[3] The initial learning or conditioning is reinforced by the action of nicotine through the brain's reward system, thus making continued use more probable. Continued use leads to continued reinforcement which leads to further use which leads to addiction. The addict's brain has become conditioned to depend upon the action of nicotine and thereby continued use is necessary to be "normal."

Genetic factors are known to predispose individuals to addiction. Studies of monozygotic twins and families with a history of drug addictions have found suggested specific genes abnormalities and alcohol-related pathological release of brain rewarding chemicals associated with alcoholism.[4] While such studies of nicotine addiction have not yet been done, it is possible that nicotine and other addictions will share common genetic biases, environmental features, *or involve in utero genetic interaction.* Mental illness may also place these persons at higher risk to seek out and become dependent upon mind altering substances.

NEUROBIOLOGY OF NICOTINE ADDICTION

The neurobiological process of nicotine addiction is similar to that of other drugs and involves an area of the brain known as the medial forebrain bundle (MFB). This is the reward system of the brain. The structures of the MFB are the frontal cortex, the nucleus accumbens (NA) and the ventral tegmental area (VTA). Nerve fibers running from the VTA to the NA are known as the mesolimbic dopaminergic pathway. These nerves release dopamine in the NA. Dopamine is a neurotransmitter which excites neurons in the NA generating the drive to repeat the brain reward through eating[5] drinking[6] and sex.[7] The natural drives: eating, drinking and copulation produce this positive reinforcement (i.e., brain reward) encouraging continuation of that behavior.

Most if not all drugs of abuse stimulate dopamine transmission in the nucleus accumbens, sustain self-administration, increase preferentially levels of extracellular dopamine and energy metabolism in the shell of the nucleus accumbens. Nicotine produces neurochemical effects in the shell that resemble closely those of cocaine and other addicting drugs. Recently reported results[8] show that the ability of nicotine to increase extracelluar dopamine in the nucleus accumbens is the result of specific activation of the mesolimbic dopaminergic neurons projecting to the shell. Nicotine interacts with the brain's dopamine system through nicotinic cholinoceptors located on both the cell bodies and terminals of dopamine neurons. Acute administration of nicotine leads to an increase in the activity of midbrain dopamine neurons as well as an increase in the release of dopamine in terminal areas. Chronic administration of nicotine results in increased binding of (3H)L-nicotine in rodent brain and this has been shown in the brains of chronic tobacco smokers as well. There are some theoretical and animal data that would support the hypothesis that endogenous opioid peptides play a role in nicotine dependence and withdrawal. Nicotine increases plasma B-endorphin-like immunoreactivity in the rat and in smokers.[9] Nicotine also increases the release of plasma levels of enkephalins.[10,11]

The idea is that an addictive drug will stimulate a reward in the brain leading to compulsive use (i.e., continued self-administration). Compulsive use should not be confused with repetitive use. The distinctive feature of compulsive use is use of the drug despite known harmful consequences.[12] Elaborate punishment paradigms have been studied which clearly show that the acute effects of drugs, the rewarding effects, are not mitigated by punishment. Just as many alcoholics will drink and vomit as long as alcohol-induced brain reward continues, smokers will smoke immediately post-op or smoke and cough. Smokers continue to smoke and recognize that clear evidence exists that smoking increases risk of cancer, stroke and cardiovascular disease. Many reports document that smokers continue to smoke even after coronary bypass surgery, cancer chemotherapy, PTCA, organ transplantation and throughout the course of conditions like COPD, asthma, and angina.

LONG-TERM EFFECTS OF DRUGS ON BRAIN FUNCTION

One new area of investigations is the role of persistent deficits produced by drug-related effects. The optimistic assertions that illicit drug use could be discontinued and the user would be able to return to normal is at odds with developmental theories which would assert that drug intoxication and addiction might interfere with normal development and further that drugs taken for their specific effects and target in the brain appear equally proficient at inducing changes in heart and other vital organs. Cocaine use is associated with increases in blood pressure which is much greater in small vessels in brain and increases the oxygen demands on the heart but decreases the available blood. Ischemic cerebrovascular accidents occur commonly in cocaine users and their significance extends beyond the PET scan deficits reported for addicts to persistent neuropsychological deficits. Abstinence may simply allow certain addicts to recognize that they can not function at their pre-morbid level or that they can not hit a curve ball as they did before cocaine. Volkow[13] has reported that cocaine causes a decrease in the number of D2 receptors with corresponding decreases in brain metabolism especially in the frontal cortex. These

drug-induced changes apparently persist for many months after abstinence. Such changes could underlie craving or the perception that the
addict would be better, would feel and think better, if they only had their
drug to use. The more cocaine use the more dopamine is released and
available to act at DA receptors but the greater the need for animals to
electrically self-stimulate pleasure systems when cocaine is no longer
available. Similar findings suggesting acute and persisting anhedonia on
withdrawal have been reported by Weiss for cocaine, alcohol, nicotine,
and opiates.[14] Once changes occur in neurotrophin, neurofilaments, gluta-
mate receptors and glial filaments use becomes addiction as brains are
changed and trained. Exposure to conditioned cues, stress, D2 agonists
and so on all make use more likely and driven. Cocaine-related ischemia
strokes and gross anatomical changes and also more subtle ventral tegmental, nucleus accumbens cell and nuclear program changes produce
neurotoxic consequences which may suggest that any short-term treatment
approach is questionable with long-term abstinence assumed to be necessary for full return to pre-morbid functioning. Changes in the brain are
both acute and prolonged and in some patients may be permanent. While
less research has been done in this area with nicotine, other similarities
between nicotine and drugs like cocaine suggest that these long-term
changes may also occur for nicotine.

TREATMENT OF ACUTE NICOTINE WITHDRAWAL

Nicotine dependence causes changes in brain function gradually over
time in response to prolonged periods of nicotine exposure. Gradual in
becoming fixed in the brain, changes persist for extended periods of time
after discontinuation of chronic nicotine administration. The more rapid
onset of nicotine effects with cigarette smoking leads to a more intensive
habit pattern that is more difficult to give up because of the frequency and
rapidity of reinforcement and the greater physical dependence on nicotine.
DSM-IV recognizes a specific nicotine withdrawal syndrome involving
dysphoric or depressed mood, insomnia, irritability, frustration, or anger,
anxiety, difficulty concentrating, restlessness, decreased heart rate and
increased appetite or weight gain. In individuals who smoke cigarettes,
heart rate decreases by 5 to 12 beats per minute in the first few days after
stopping smoking, and weight increases an average of 2-3 kg over the first
year after stopping smoking. Mild symptoms of withdrawal may occur
after switching to low-tar/nicotine cigarettes and after stopping the use of
smokeless (chewing) tobacco, nicotine gum, or nicotine patches.
Withdrawal symptoms can begin within a few hours of cessation, typi-

cally peak in 1-4 days, and last for 3-4 weeks. Nicotine withdrawal includes a desire for sweets and impaired performance on tasks requiring vigilance. In comparisons to other drug withdrawal states, nicotine withdrawal has a time course similar to alcohol or heroin but without the extremes of DTs, vomiting and so forth. Nicotine remains among the very most addictive of drugs.[15] Some smokers will experience greater withdrawal distress from nicotine than some addicts experience from cessation of opioids or other drugs. Supporting this view is our experience that alcoholics who smoke prefer to detoxify from alcohol and remain smokers and not vice versa. Nicotine withdrawal appears to have hunger, weight gain and nicotine craving as prominent protracted withdrawal symptoms.[16] Untreated subtle, non-nicotine withdrawal of smokers may be a cause of relapse and suggests that we have such an incomplete view of the neurobiology of withdrawal that treatment for any withdrawal state is at best partial.

Nicotine withdrawal has been studied in animals allowing us to follow changes in important brain regions during drug self-administration and absence. Again, the actions of nicotine on the brain's dopamine system are thought to play a critical role in its behavioral effects and ability to produce dependence. The effects of withdrawal from chronic nicotine exposure on the dopamine system have recently been studied.[17] They examine the activity of substantia nigra (A9) and ventral tegmental area (A10) dopamine cells in rats undergoing spontaneous withdrawal from chronic nicotine administration. Chronic administration of nicotine led to a decreased firing rate of A10 but not A9 dopamine cells. Upon withdrawal A10 firing returned to control levels but A9 dopamine cells significantly increased over control levels. A rebound in dopamine activity upon withdrawal may suggest a dysregulation in these important motivational and mood systems.

TREATMENT OF NICOTINE ADDICTION/DEPENDENCE

In attempting to define a treatment program for nicotine or other drug dependence, one must first come to some understanding as to the treatment goal. O'Brien and McLellan have suggested that almost everyone has a friend or relative who has been in treatment for a tobacco, alcohol or other drug dependence and has relapsed.[18] This has suggested to many Americans that addiction treatment is unsuccessful. However, "cure," per se, is unrealistic for most chronic diseases. As with other chronic illnesses, continued treatment, prolonging a remission and improving the patient's health and quality of life are more realistic goals.

While often thought of as less serious or addictive than other drugs, nicotine dependence is especially resistant to treatment interventions. Research on treatment programs indicates a success rate of approximately 50% for Alcoholism treatment, 60% for opioid dependence and 55% for cocaine. However, the success rate for nicotine dependence is only 30%. Thus, nicotine is the addicting drug that has the poorest success rate with only 20-30% of users not returning to smoking at 12 months after treatment. Of those who successfully quit, less than 25% quit on their first attempt. Most individuals who smoke have 3-4 failures before they stop smoking for good. In the United States, about 45% of those who have ever smoked eventually stop smoking. Although over 80% of individuals who smoke express a desire to stop smoking and 35% try to stop each year, less than 5% are successful in unaided attempts to quit.

Nicotine Replacement Therapy

Nicotine replacement and detoxification is frequently prescribed as part of a smoking cessation program. The first generally available nicotine replacement was nicotine chewing gum. However, oral and gastric side-effects impaired absorption when taken with coffee or other beverages. Some patients apparently transferred nicotine dependency from cigarettes to the gum.[19] After nicotine gum other replacement transdermal patches, intranasal sprays and inhalers have been tried. A recent meta-analysis on efficacy of nicotine replacement therapies in smoking cessation[20] from nearly 18,000 subjects from all randomized trials of nicotine gum, patches, sprays and inhalers has strongly suggested that all of the currently available forms of nicotine replacement are effective therapies to aid smoking cessation.

There does exist some controversy as to how much nicotine and for how long is ideal.[21] Dale[22] found that the 22 mg patches under-dose the majority of smokers and higher doses are safe, providing better withdrawal relief and increased treatment outcome efficacy. Higher dose nicotine gum is more effective than low dose and some have found that nicotine gum helps patients on the patch. Jorenby[23] showed no long-term outcome differences between 22 and 44 mg patch doses although short-term effects were better with the 44 mg dose. Higher nicotine replacement doses, tailoring treatment, or adding behavior therapy to nicotine patch therapy don't necessarily increase quit rates above the rates reported for the patch alone. Treatment with nicotine remains cost effective despite its limitations.[24] The patch is twice as cost-effective as the 2 mg gum but equal to the 4 mg gum. The physician can further increase cost effectiveness by prescribing a 2 week supply of the patch with a recommendation that patients not refill their prescriptions if they smoke during the first 2 week period. This strategy improves cost effectiveness by 25% but overall one year smoking relapse rates are 70-80%. Newer treatments are coming from clinical trials to the clinics such as the nicotine inhaler and nasal sprays. Nasal administration systems have been developed to mimic cigarette smoking producing venous plasma concentrations of 5-12 µg/liter. Venous plasma concentrations produced by the spray are lower than those produced by smoking (inhaled nicotine reaches the brain in 7 seconds via arterial boli and venous blood nicotine concentrations peak in 5 minutes) and the rise to peak is also slower than produced by smoking.[25] Using inhaler allowed weaning from smoking in 17% of patients vs. placebo rate of 9% at 6 months and 13% vs. placebo at 8% at one year. Subjects averaged six inhalers a day with side effects including throat and mouth irritation and cough.[26]

For the most part, these nicotine replacement therapies appear to be relatively safe. *Smoking* is the problem not nicotine. Smoking tobacco increases the risk of lung cancer, bladder cancer and cardiovascular disease and has been described as a major public health problem. Nicotine has been related to tobacco's stimulatory effects and dependence liability but it is unclear what role if any it plays in negative health consequences. A recent two year study[27] of long-term inhalation of nicotine in rats failed to find any increase in mortality or atherosclerosis or increased tumors. No microscopic or macroscopic lung tumors or increase in pulmonary neuroendocrine cells were found. The only finding was a reduced body weight. This study failed to find any harmful effects of nicotine when given alone. Further studies are necessary but it is logical to assume from the release of nicotine preparations like gum, the patch and inhalers are safe and that the major health risks are in the smoke, the delivery rather than in the nicotine.

TREATMENT FAILURE AND RELAPSE

The high rates of relapse after nicotine detoxification must not be considered treatment failure given the above stated goals for drug dependence. In addition, the dirth of viable non-detoxification and abstinence approaches to treatment makes all patients fit into one treatment rather than have competing viable treatment approaches for patients. Relapse should be considered no more a failure than a high glucose could be considered treatment failure by an endocrinologist. It is merely a hurdle to overcome and even to be expected. Likewise, compliance with any long-term therapy is an important issue to consider. The daily chore of complying with medication regimens for addiction is as problematic as taking daily injections of insulin is for diabetics. Non-compliance is obviously directly related to relapse in addicts and medical morbidity in diabetics. Relapse is part of the addictive disease and imperfect current approaches to treatment. We need to educate addicts as diligently as we would any other person with a chronic illness. They need continuous support and respect as persons with a chronic medical disease. Considering addiction or addiction treatment relapse a moral failure is as ridiculous as considering overweight, cardiovascular disease, cancer of all forms, or diabetes the result of moral failure.[28]

Compulsive drug seeking is the result of a progressive and persistent hypersensitivity of specific neural systems induced in susceptible individuals by the intermittent drug use. Neural sensitization can more than double the original effect of the drug and is the opposite of drug tolerance or reduced responsiveness. The neural systems sensitized by drugs mediate specific motivational processes that cause the act to become attractive or sought after. This process that cause the perception of the event to over-focus on drugs and drug stimuli that they call wanting. Repeated drug use sensitizes neural substrates of wanting–want drugs more and enjoy them less. Unconscious wanting becomes a reflex activation not always accessible to consciousness. People want all kinds of things without knowing why. Relapse is logical in this context and can be treated once we understand its neurobiology and genesis. People are not directly aware of wanting and liking. Drug self administration in the absence of self reported craving supports the notion that drug use becomes automatic or decoupled from conscious control. This could occur through sensitized incentive salience acquired through associative pairing of neural hyperactivity with the act of drug use or through compulsive repetition of the act itself. Biological treatments may be especially helpful in the treatment of relapse.

Knowledge of and treatment of premorbid or concurrent psychiatric illness, such as major depression, manic-depression, eating or panic/anxiety disorders, helps to cope with the double trouble of comorbidity and may reduce relapse and treatment failure.[29] Nicotine dependence is more common among patients who are depressed or have a family history of depression. Patients who have increased depression on smoking discontinuation are also more likely to relapse. Nicotine dependence and smoking may be an early marker for another addiction such as alcoholism. Clinical trials with antidepressants and Naltrexone have added considerably to our understanding of tobacco smoking or nicotine dependence. The experimental use of these agents to reduce relapse is also supported by recent data exploring the differences between nicotine administration and smoking on brain MAO and other activity as measured by Positron Emission Tomography. Comorbid addictive illness is common as is the practice of shifting drugs depending on availability. Nicotine can temporarily satisfy an opiate or cocaine addict or alcoholic. Nicotine dependence is commonly comorbid with alcoholism. Nicotine can serve as a positive reinforcer for rats, taking the place of cocaine on a temporary basis. In man, drinking and smoking seem commonplace and persistent. Smokers with active alcoholism in the preceding year were 60% less likely to quit than were smokers with no history of alcoholism. In contrast, smokers whose alcoholism had remitted were at least as likely to quit as smokers with no history of alcoholism. Remission of alcoholism was associated with more than a threefold increase in the likelihood of subsequent smoking cessation.[30] Discontinuation of alcoholism is a good strategy to increase success in smoking cessation. Abstinence from all drugs of abuse and treatment for all drug dependencies should be encouraged.

TREATMENT

There are three general phases to the treatment of addiction. While these stages have been applied to alcoholism and other addictions, they should be vigorously applied to people smoking cigarettes and addicted to nicotine. The first phase is Getting Started, the process of developing the willingness to enter treatment, or what Alcoholics Anonymous calls "the desire" to stop smoking, drinking and using drugs. Physicians help patients with their resistance by simply asking about smoking, describing health consequences and risks in them and offering to help. There are many important roles for society and health professionals in this first phase of the addiction treatment experience, including decreasing social tolerance for the use of tobacco products, reducing second hand smoke exposure, elimination of public indoor smoking, and providing incentives for stopping. The second phase of addiction treatment is Stopping Use, which can be done either on an inpatient or an outpatient basis. For smokers, this involves choosing a quit date and stopping smoking. It is in this stage that medical treatment of abstinence is important. This is where organized, medically managed detoxification takes place. It is here that nicotine replacement therapies can help avoid a relapse to smoking behavior. Physicians should consider all approaches which help the patient succeed in detoxification where they have failed before. The third phase of addiction treatment is Staying Clean and Sober. This is where relapse prevention and the 12-step programs, Alcoholics Anonymous, Narcotics

Anonymous, Al-Anon, and other programs built on the original founda-
tions of AA, play their biggest roles. Unfortunately, they have not been
applied with as much vigor in smokers. Relapse-preventing psychopharmacology is an important new addition to this phase.

Medications which deny brain reward access to rewarding drugs of
abuse rather than punish the addict for using are in the early phases of a
dramatic change in the field of Addiction Medicine and Addiction Psychiatry. Treatment with the opiate antagonist Naltrexone has made some
relapsing, and even chronic relapsing, alcoholics more amenable to 12-step
fellowships and behavior change. Acamprosate is reported to have similar
effects through an independent mechanism in treatment trials in Europe.
Naltrexone can prevent relapse in addictive illnesses as apparently diverse
as alcoholism and heroin addiction. While Naltrexone may also prevent
relapse in cigarette smokers, the data reported to date does not thoroughly
support such a statement.[31,32] However, we have observed in the course of
treating opiate addicts and more recently alcoholics with Naltrexone that
smoking can become less compelling and abstinence more likely. In addition, we have evidence from preliminary data that Naltrexone can safely
and effectively increase the success of nicotine detoxification treatments
as measured by a significantly reduced relapse rate in a random assignment placebo controlled double-blind study. These data are supported by
research that shows that morphine reverses nicotine abstinence and Naloxone provokes immediate abstinence in nicotine dependent mice.[33] Naloxone also interferes with nicotine alleviation of the nicotine abstinence
syndrome.[34] A rodent model of nicotine abstinence syndrome using continuous subcutaneous infusion of nicotine tartrate and spontaneous behavioral signs which emerge after discontinuation of administration or injection of nicotinic antagonist mecamylamine demonstrated that the nicotine
abstinence signs resemble those observed in opiate withdrawal. Again,
these results support the hypothesis that endogenous opioid peptides play
a role in nicotine dependence and withdrawal. Naturally, as nicotine withdrawal more closely resembles opiate withdrawal, treatment for acute
abstinence with Clonidine and prevention of relapse with Naltrexone become all the more theoretically appealing.

Research and much clinical experience over the past several years
clearly demonstrates that the process of addiction involves much more
than the addict continuing use to prevent withdrawal. Motivational changes
described by the addict as wanting to use, missing the high, preferring the
high to "normal state" and the glamorization and psuedodrama of the
addict life conspire to make reinitiating of use part of an overall rational-
ization that this time use will be limited and controlled. Positive reinforce-

ment alone is enough to initiate and maintain addiction. The fact that so many addicts relapse well past detoxification and any influence of withdrawal indicates that the physical dependence model of addiction is alone inadequate. This fact also raises the possibility that the motivational changes are related to long-term or even permanent shifts in brain function in mesolimbic and frontal areas which are relatively silent but which can bias thinking toward reinitiating use.

Research with other drugs indicates that the best treatment outcomes involve more than detoxification and focus on drug replacement relapse prevention, and in some cases long-term residential care. This was based on the finding that while the drug was long gone, persistent social and psychological deficits required intensive care from facilities such as Phoenix House and Daytop. Again, superior success rates with some of the most apparently disabled addicts were reported and correlated with length of time in treatment. For opiate dependence the treatment options include detoxification and abstinence but also numerous other more powerful approaches including Narcotic Anonymous, Residential Treatment Centers, Day Programs, methadone, buprenorphine, naltrexone, and so on. Unfortunately, tobacco smoking disorders have been trivialized to the point that maintenance, residential and other long-term treatments have not been advocated. The more we think of them as nicotine dependence the more the tendency is to try to fit all of the patients into detoxification and abstinence. What could be the down-side of treating chronically relapsing smokers with years of nicotine replacement?

While we develop better treatments it is important to remember that Prevention is the single most effective treatment for addictive disorders.[35] The increasing trend of cigarette and marijuana smoking among teenagers bodes ill for our nation's future health. Our first priority must be to prevent first use, and educate the public about addiction and the health consequences of smoking.

CONCLUSION

Addiction is a chronic medical disorder which is best treated with relapse prevention in clear view as a desired outcome. Addictions are chronic disorders not acute conditions like a broken leg. Addiction does not end when the drug is removed from the body (detoxification) or when the acute post drug-taking illness dissipates (withdrawal). Rather, the underlying addictive disorder persists, and this persistence produces a tendency to relapse to active drug taking. Detoxification does not address the underlying disorder and thus is not adequate treatment.[36] While we have made substantial progress in the acute treatment of withdrawal, the ease or success of withdrawal has little to do with the success of treatment or relapse. Focusing on the changes induced by drugs which makes relapse more likely than abstinence has led to brain research and new pharmacological treatments.

Drug addiction is a brain disease and new treatments are being tested which help prevent relapse, reverse changes induced by the drugs, and even prevent re-intoxication. The application of these new treatments requires a re-education of treatment professionals so that patients with addiction can benefit from combined treatment in the same way that depressed patients are treated–medications plus therapy is better than either alone. Naltrexone has been shown to improve treatment outcome. Medication as a primary modality is limited by compliance but the actual data shows clearly that active psychosocial treatment plus Naltrexone is better than Naltrexone or active psychosocial treatment alone.[37] Addiction is a life long chronic relapsing illness from which there is no specific cure. Treatment should be individualized as much as possible and still retain the essential ingredients shown to be effective in the past.

While we develop better treatments it is important to remember that Prevention is the single most effective treatment for addictive disorders. The increasing trend of cigarette and marijuana smoking among teenagers bodes ill for our nation's future health. Our first priority must be to prevent first use, and educate the public about addiction and the health consequences of smoking.

REFERENCES

1. Benowitz NL. Cigarette Smoking and Nicotine Addiction. The Medical Clinics of North America. 76.2:415-437, 1992.

2. Gold MS. Is there a treatment or treatments for drug abuse or addiction? Contemporary Psychology 38:1119-1120, 1993.

3. Wonnacott S. The relevance of receptor binding studies to tobacco research. British Journal of Addiction 86:537-541, 1991.

4. Noble, EP. The D2 dopamine receptor gene: a review of association studies in alcoholism. Behav Genet 23(2):199-29, 1993 Mar.

5. Radhakishun FS, et al. Scheduled eating increases dopamine release in the nucleus accumbens of food deprived rats as assessed with on-line micro dialysis. Neuroscience Letter 85:351-356, 1988.

6. Chang VC, et al. Extracellular dopamine increase in the nucleus accumbens following rehydration or sodium repletion in rats. Soc. Neuroscience Abstr. 14:527, 1988.

7. Goldstein A. Addictive Drugs and the Brain. Addiction: From biology to drug policy. New York: W.H. Freeman, 1994. 53-59.

8. Pontieri FE, Tanda G, Orzi F, DiChiara G. Effects of nicotine on the nucleus accumbens and similarity to those of addictive drugs. Nature 382: 255-257, 1996.

9. Gilbert DG, Meliska CJ, Williams CL, Jensen RA. Subjective correlates of cigarette-induced elevations of beta-endorphin and cortisol. Psychopharmacology 106:275-281, 1992.

10. Pomerleau OF, Fertig JB, Seyler E, Jaffe J. Neuroendocrine reactivity to nicotine in smokers. Psychopharmacology 81:61-67, 1983.

11. Houdi AA, Pierzchala K, Marson L, Palkovits M, Van Loon GR. Nicotine-induced alteration of Tyr-Gly Gly and Met-enkepahlin neuron activity. Peptides 12:161-161, 1991.

12. Ibid.

13. Volkow, National Academy of Science, 7/29/96, Washington DC.

14. Weiss, National Academy of Science, 7/29/96, Washington DC.

15. Hughes JR. The nicotine withdrawal syndrome: A brief review and update, International Journal of Smoking Cessation, 1:21-26, 1992.

16. Hughes JR. Protracted Withdrawal, Am J Psychiatry 151:785-786, 1994.

17. Rasmussen K, Czachura JF. Nicotine withdrawal leads to increased firing rates of midbrain dopamine neurons. NeuroReport 7:329-332, 1995.

18. O'Brien CP, McLellan, AT. Myths about the treatment of addiction. Lancet 347:237-240, 1996.

19. Hughes JR, Hatsukami DK, Skoog KP. Physical dependence on nicotine in gum. JAMA 255:3277-3279, 1986.

20. Silagy C, Man D, Fowler G, Lodge M. Met-analysis on efficacy of nicotine replacement therapies in smoking cessation. Lancet 343:139-142, 1994.

21. Hughes JR. Treatment of nicotine dependence: Is more better? JAMA 274:1390-1391, 1995.

22. Dale LC, Hurt RD, Offord KP, Lawson GM, Croghan IT, Schroeder DR. High-dose nicotine patch therapy: percentage of replacement and smoking cessation. JAMA:54:98-106,1993.

23. Jorenby DE, Smith SS Fiore MC. et al. Varying nicotine patch dose and type of smoking cessation counseling, JAMA 274:1347-1352, 1995.

24. Fiscella K, Franks P. Cost-effectiveness of the transdermal nicotine patch as an adjunct to physicians' smoking cessation counseling, JAMA 275:1247-1251, 1996.

25. Schneider NG, Lunell E, Olmstead RE, Fagerstrom KO. Clinical pharmacokinetics of nasal nicotine delivery. Clin Pharmacokinet 1:65-80, 1996.

26. Schneider NG, Olmstead R, Nilsson F, Mody VF, Franzon M, Doan K. Efficacy of a nicotine inhaler in smoking cessation: a double-blind, placebo-controlled trial. Addiction 91:1293-1306, 1996.

27. Waldrum HL, Nilsen OG, Nilsen T, Rorvik H, Syversen U, Sandvik AK, Haugen OA, Torp SH, Brenna E. Long-term effects of inhaled nicotine. Life Sciences 58:1339-1346, 1996.

28. O'Brien CP, McLellan AT. Myths about the treatment of addiction. Lancet. 347:237-240, 1996.

29. Gold MS, Miller NS. The biology of Addictive and Psychiatric Disorders in Treating Coexisting Psychiatric and Addictive Disorders, Miller, NS (Ed.) Hazelden, 1994 pp 35-52.

30. Breslau N, Peterson E, Schultz L, Andreski P, Chilcoat H. Are smokers with alcohol disorders less likely to quit? Am J Public Health 86:985-990, 1996.

31. Gorelick DA, Rose J, Jarvik ME. Effect of naloxone on cigarette smoking. J Subst. Abuse 1:153-159, 1989.

32. Karras A, Kane JM. Naloxone reduces cigarette smoking. Life Sciences 27:1541-1545, 1980.

33. Malin DH, Lake JR, Payne MC, Short PE, Carter VA, Cunningham JS, Wilson OB. Nicotine alleviation of nicotine abstinence syndrome is naloxone reversible. Pharmacol Biochem Beh 53:81-85, 1996.

34. Gold MS. Overview: Role of the Physician, Prevention of Addictive Disorders, Section III, Chapter 1, American Society of Addiction Medicine's (ASAM) first official Manual of Addiction Medicine, Principles of Addiction Medicine, ASAM, Chevy Chase, Maryland, 1994.

35. O'Brien CP, McLellan AT. Myths about the treatment of addiction. Lancet 347:237-240, 1996.

36. Volpicelli JR, Volpicelli LA, O'Brien CP. Medical management of alcohol dependence: Clinical use and limitations of naltrexone treatment. Alcohol & Alcoholism 30:789-798, 1995.

37. Gold MS. Neurobiology of addiction and recovery: The brain, the drive for the drug and the 12-Step Fellowship. J Substance Abuse Treatment 11(2):93-97, 1994.

Neuropharmacological Actions of Cigarette Smoke: Brain Monoamine Oxidase B (MAO B) Inhibition

J. S. Fowler, PhD
N. D. Volkow, MD
G.-J. Wang, MD
N. Pappas, MS
J. Logan, PhD
R. MacGregor, BS
D. Alexoff, BA
A. P. Wolf, PhD
D. Warner, AA
R. Cilento, MD
I. Zezulkova, MD

J. S. Fowler, N. D. Volkow, G.-J. Wang, N. Pappas, J. Logan, R. MacGregor, D. Alexoff, A. P. Wolf, D. Warner, R. Cilento and I. Zezulkova are all affiliated with the Chemistry and Medical Departments, Brookhaven National Laboratory, Upton, NY. N. D. Volkow is also affiliated with the Department of Psychiatry, State University of New York at Stony Brook, Stony Brook, NY.

Address correspondence to: J. S. Fowler, Department of Chemistry and Medicine, Brookhaven National Laboratory, Upton, NY 11973.

The authors are grateful to Richard Ferrieri, Robert Carciello, Colleen Shea, Noelwah Netusil, Kathy Pascani, Carol Redvanly, Payton King and Lois Caligiuri for their assistance in various parts of this study and John Gatley, David Schlyer, Robert Hitzemann, Richard Setlow and Carol Creutz for helpful discussions. They are also grateful to the subjects who participated in this study.

This research was carried out at Brookhaven National Laboratory (BNL) under contract DE-AC02-76CH00016 with the U. S. Department of Energy and supported by its Office of Health and Environmental Research and by National Institutes of Health grant NS 15380 and DA 06891.

[Haworth co-indexing entry note]: "Neuropharmacological Actions of Cigarette Smoke: Brain Monoamine Oxidase B (MAO B) Inhibition." Fowler, J. S. et al. Co-published simultaneously in *Journal of Addictive Diseases* (The Haworth Medical Press, an imprint of The Haworth Press, Inc.) Vol. 17, No. 1, 1998, pp. 23-34; and: *Smoking and Illicit Drug Use* (ed: Mark S. Gold, and Barry Stimmel) The Haworth Medical Press, an imprint of The Haworth Press, Inc., 1998, pp. 23-34. Single or multiple copies of this article are available for a fee from The Haworth Document Delivery Service [1-800-342-9678, 9:00 a.m. - 5:00 p.m. (EST). E-mail address: getinfo@haworth.com].

SUMMARY. We measured the concentration of brain monoamine oxidase B (MAO B; EC 1.4.3.4) in 8 smokers and compared it with that in 8 non-smokers and in 4 former smokers using positron emission tomography (PET) and deuterium substituted [^{11}C]L-deprenyl ([^{11}C]L-deprenyl-D2) as a radiotracer for MAO B. Smokers had significantly lower brain MAO B than non-smokers as measured by the model term λk_3 which is a function of MAO B activity. Reductions were observed in all brain regions. Low brain MAO B in the cigarette smoker appears to be a pharmacological rather than a genetic effect since former smokers did not differ from non-smokers. Brain MAO B inhibition by cigarette smoke is of relevance in light of the inverse association between smoking and Parkinson's disease and a high prevalence of smoking in psychiatric disorders and in substance abuse. Though nicotine is at the core of the neuropharmacological actions of tobacco smoke, MAO B inhibition may also be an important variable in understanding and treating tobacco smoke addiction. *[Article copies available for a fee from The Haworth Document Delivery Service: 1-800-342-9678. E-mail address: getinfo@ haworth.com]*

In spite of the fact that 45 million persons in the United States regularly smoke cigarettes, there is relatively little known about the neuropharmacological effects of cigarette smoke on the brain, apart from the effects of nicotine.[1] This is of particular relevance considering that smoking accounts for 400,000 deaths per year in the United States (more than 60 times the number related to heroin and cocaine use) and 50% of smokers who suffer a major illness related to tobacco smoke exposure are unable to stop smoking.[1,2,3] Other aspects of cigarette smoking which merit attention are reports of a negative association between smoking and the development of Parkinson's[4,5] and the prevalence of cigarette smoking among patients with psychiatric disorders[6,7] and addiction to other substances[8] compared to the population at large. These reports highlight the importance of understanding the neuropharmacological effects of cigarette smoking which contribute both to smoking behavior and to smoking epidemiology.

MAO is a flavin containing enzyme which exists in two subtypes (A and B) and metabolizes neurotransmitter amines such as dopamine, norepinephrine and serotonin producing hydrogen peroxide as a by-product.[9] Reports that cigarette smokers have low platelet MAO[10,11,12,13] and that exposure of animals to cigarette smoke inhibits MAO[12,14,15,16] have led to the proposal that chemical substances in cigarette smoke which inhibit MAO contribute to some of its pharmacological actions.[17] However, the effects of exposure to tobacco smoke on MAO B in living human brain have not been measured.

We have developed deuterium substituted [^{11}C]L-deprenyl ([^{11}C]L-deprenyl-D2) as a radiotracer for measuring MAO B in the living human brain using PET.[18] We summarize here the results of a recent study comparing brain MAO B in smokers, non-smokers and former smokers using [^{11}C]L-deprenyl-D2.[19]

MATERIALS AND METHODS

Subjects

These studies followed the guidelines of the Human Subjects Research Committee at Brookhaven National Laboratory and informed consent was obtained from each subject. Eight current cigarette smokers (6 males and 2 females, age range 23-62; average 44 ± 14 years) who smoked from 0.5-2.5 packs of cigarettes a day for at least 3 years volunteered for this study. A group of 8 subjects (5 males and 3 females, age range 27-67 years; average 46 ± 14 years) with no smoking history and four subjects (males, age range 43-86; average 61 ± 19 years) who had quit smoking at least 7 years prior to this study were studied for comparison. Subjects were free from neurologic, psychiatric and cardiovascular disease and were free of medication except for one of the smokers who was receiving 1 aspirin/ day and cardizem (480 mg/day) for treatment of hypertension. Subjects with a past or present history of drug abuse (except nicotine as described, and caffeine) were excluded. Smokers refrained from smoking during the entire PET study and were scanned 1.7-12 hours after the last cigarette.

PET Procedure

Each of the subjects had one PET scan with [^{11}C]L- deprenyl-D2 using a CTI 931 tomograph (6 × 6 × 6.5 mm, full width half maximum, 15 slices, Computer Technologies Inc., CTI 931) following the procedure described previously.[18,20] Sequential PET scans were obtained immediately after injection for a total of 60 minutes with the following timing: 10 × 1 min frames; 4 × 5 min frames; 3 × 10 min frames. An arterial plasma input function for [^{11}C]L-deprenyl-D2 was also measured as described.[21] Brain glucose metabolism was also measured in 15 of the subjects with [18]FDG as previously described.[22] All PET studies were carried out in a quiet, dimly lit room with eyes open and ears unoccluded.

Image Analysis

Regions of interest were drawn directly on PET scans. For the purpose of region identification, we added the images obtained from 30 to 60 minutes after tracer injection. A template that used as a reference the brain atlas of Matsui and Hirano[23] was projected into the "averaged" PET image and manually fitted for appropriate neuroanatomical location. Regions of interest for the following brain areas were obtained: occipital cortex, frontal cortex, cingulate gyrus, parietal cortex, temporal cortex, pons, thalamus, basal ganglia, and cerebellum. Regions were identified in at least two contiguous slices and the weighted average was obtained for each region. In addition, an approximate measure for the whole brain (global) was obtained by averaging radioactivity concentrations in the 6 central slices. The regions were then projected to the dynamic scans to obtain time-activity curves. In the subjects in whom both MAO B (with [^{11}C]L-deprenyl-D2) and brain glucose metabolism (with ^{18}FDG) were measured, brain regions from the [^{11}C]L-deprenyl-D2 scans were projected onto the ^{18}FDG scans with slight adjustments made for re-positioning.

Data Analysis

For each subject, PET time-activity data from different brain regions along with time-activity data for [^{11}C]L-deprenyl-D2 in arterial plasma were used to calculate the model term Ki, a kinetic constant which determines the rate of trapping of [^{11}C]L-deprenyl-D2 (which is a function of both the concentration of MAO B and blood flow) and K_1, the blood to tissue transport constant. An approximate blood volume correction (4%) was subtracted from the PET data prior to parameter optimization. K_1 is related to blood flow (F) through the following equation.[24]

$$K_1 = F(1 - e^{-(PS/F)}) \qquad \text{(eq 1)}$$

where PS is the permeability-surface area product. Assuming a three-compartment model which allows for both the transport and trapping of ligand, Ki can be written as

$$Ki = K_1 k_3 / (k_2 + k_3) = K_1 \lambda k_3 / (K_1 + \lambda k_3) \qquad \text{(eq 2)}$$

where k_2 is the tissue to plasma efflux constant and k_3 is proportional to the concentration of MAO B. Ki is also written in terms of the product λk_3 which is independent of blood flow ($\lambda = K_1/k_2$)[25] but is a more robust parameter than k_3.[26] λk_3 can be calculated from equation 2 if Ki and K_1 are known.

Ki was obtained graphically from a transformation of plasma and tissue time-activity data.[27] Ki was taken as the average of slopes from 6 to 45 and from 6 to 55 minutes. The initial time was taken as the time from which linearity was observed. K_1 was calculated using a rearrangement method.[28] In this method the tissue radioactivity, region of interest (*ROI*) and plasma radioactivity, *Cp* are related to model parameters as given by

$$ROI(T) = K_1 \int_0^T Cp(t)dt + K_1 k_3 \int_0^T \int_0^t Cp(t')dt - (k_2 + k_3) \int_0^T ROI(t)dt$$

Using *Ki* from eq (2), this can be rearranged to give

$$ROI(T) = K_1 \int_0^T Cp(t)dt + (k_2 + k_3)(Ki \int_0^T \int_0^t Cp(t')dt' \ dt - \int_0^T ROI(t)dt)$$

This is a bilinear regression with coefficients K_1 and $k_2 + k_3$ computed using standard methods.[29]

Brain glucose metabolism (*LCMRglu* expressed as μmol glucose/100 g brain/minute) was calculated as described previously.[22]

Non-smokers, former smokers and smokers were compared using Student's t-test (two tail). Model terms compared were the plasma to brain transfer constant, K_1 and λk_3 which is a function of MAO B activity.

RESULTS AND DISCUSSION

The major finding from this study is that smokers have a marked reduction in brain MAO B relative to non-smokers. The model term λk_3 was reduced by about 40% in smokers compared to non-smokers (Table 1). The reduction in MAO B concentration was observed across all brain regions.

In contrast to the large decrease in λk_3, in smokers compared to non-smokers, the blood to brain transfer constant (K_1) did not differ ($p > 0.13$). This indicates that smoking does not change [11C]L-deprenyl-D2 delivery to the brain (see Table 1) and is evidence that the changes in radiotracer trapping are not due to changes in radiotracer delivery. This is consistent with the report that there is no significant difference in brain blood flow between smokers and non-smokers.[30] Figure 1 shows a comparison of K_1 and λk_3 in non-smokers, smokers and former smokers for the basal ganglia.

Fifteen of the subjects were also scanned with [18]FDG to assess the specificity of the effect. Brain glucose metabolism did not differ between

TABLE 1. Comparison of model terms K_1, and λk_3 for non-smokers (n = 8), smokers (n = 8) and former smokers (n = 4). There was no significant difference in K_1 between non-smokers, smokers and former smokers. There was a significant difference between non-smokers and smokers in λk_3 (p < 0.001) but no difference between non-smokers and former smokers.

Brain Region	K_1 $(ml_{plasma}\ (cc_{brain})^{-1}min^{-1})$			λk_3 $(cc_{brain}\ (ml_{plasma})^{-1}min^{-1})$			
	non-smokers	smokers	former smokers	non-smokers	smokers	former smokers	% difference[a]
global	0.50 ± 0.11	0.46 ± 0.09	0.42 ± 0.06	0.161 ± 0.024	0.103 ± 0.034	0.20 ± 0.04	−36
basal ganglia	0.67 ± 0.15	0.70 ± 0.14	0.59 ± 0.09	0.38 ± 0.07	0.195 ± 0.084	0.44 ± 0.07	−49
thalamus	0.82 ± 0.18	0.77 ± 0.18	0.73 ± 0.13	0.31 ± 0.065	0.18 ± 0.08	0.38 ± 0.035	−42
cerebellum	0.66 ± 0.16	0.63 ± 0.13	0.55 ± 0.03	0.15 ± 0.03	0.09 ± 0.04	0.17 ± 0.012	−40
cingulate gyrus	0.70 ± 0.15	0.62 ± 0.10	0.57 ± 0.15	0.22 ± 0.05	0.13 ± 0.05	0.25 ± 0.04	−41
frontal cortex	0.67 ± 0.14	0.59 ± 0.11	0.54 ± 0.11	0.18 ± 0.025	0.11 ± 0.05	0.21 ± 0.035	−39
occipital cortex	0.72 ± 0.23	0.70 ± 0.16	0.53 ± 0.07	0.155 ± 0.015	0.087 ± 0.04	0.20 ± 0.04	−44
pons	0.58 ± 0.20	0.55 ± 0.16	0.51 ± 0.12	0.277 ± 0.05	0.147 ± 0.071	0.31 ± 0.02	−47

a. non-smokers vs. smokers

smokers and non-smokers. The average values for the whole brain were 32.9 ± 2.1 and 33.3 ± 3.2 μmol/100g/min for the non-smokers and smokers respectively (data not shown). PET images comparing MAO B and glucose metabolism in a non-smoker and a smoker are shown in Figure 2.

Differences in MAO B between smokers and non-smokers appear to be due to pharmacological and not genetic factors as shown by normal MAO B values in former smokers (Table 1). Previous studies are also consistent with pharmacological effect of cigarette smoke. For example, though platelet MAO B is lower in cigarette smokers than in non-smokers, it returns to normal values in individuals who had stopped smoking.[11] In addition, cigarette smoke and extracts of cigarette smoke inhibit MAO both *in vivo* and *in vitro*.[12,14,15,16] Though the mechanisms of MAO inhibition by cigarette smoke are not known, it has been proposed that cyanomethylation (brought about by formaldehyde and cyanide in smoke) of the reactive amino groups in the MAO protein may reduce its catalytic activity.[17] It has been shown that nicotine does not inhibit MAO B in physiologically relevant concentrations.[10]

In this study, the time interval between last cigarette and the PET scan ranged from 1.7-12 hours. Since we do not know the time course of MAO B recovery after withdrawal from cigarettes, it is possible that we have underestimated the degree of chronic inhibition in the cigarette smoker

FIGURE 1. Comparison of average data for K_1 and λk_3 for the basal ganglia for non-smokers, smokers and former smokers. Units for K_1 are ml$_{\text{plasma}}$ (cc$_{\text{brain}}$)$^{-1}$min^{-1} and units for λk_3 are cc$_{\text{brain}}$ (ml$_{\text{plasma}}$)$^{-1}$min^{-1}).

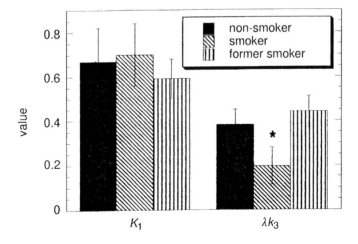

FIGURE 2. Comparison of MAO B activity as measured by [¹¹C]L-deprenyl-D2 and glucose metabolism as measured by ¹⁸FDG in a non-smoker and in a smoker at the level of the thalamus. Note that the smoker has reduced MAO B activity relative to the non-smoker but that the non-smoker and the smoker have similiar brain glucose metabolism.

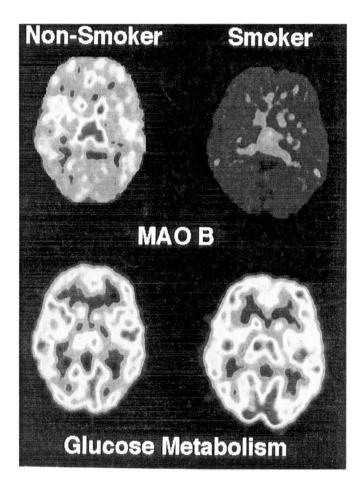

where the recycle time is one hour or less.[3] *In vitro* studies have reported that cigarette smoke irreversibly inhibits MAO.[14] If the irreversible inhibition of MAO also occurs *in vivo,* then the effects of cigarette smoking on the enzyme would be predicted to be cumulative because the synthesis rate of human brain MAO B is slow with a half-life of about 40 days.[31]

Though we do not know the relative influence of different smoking variables on the degree of MAO B inhibition, factors such as cigarette type, daily smoking dose, years of smoking, time interval between last cigarette and PET scan and smoking behavior need to be investigated.

The functional and medical consequences of long term partial inhibition of human brain MAO B are not known. However, MAO B is important in the metabolism of brain dopamine[32] and thus its inhibition by tobacco smoke would be predicted to enhance brain dopamine. This is of particular relevance since nicotine is known to activate the brain dopamine system.[33,34] Thus these two pharmacological actions of cigarette smoke, nicotine-mediated increases in dopamine activity and MAO B inhibition, may function synergistically to enhance brain dopamine. The possibility that this could compensate for age- or disease-related losses in dopaminergic neurons[35] or could enhance the dopaminergic effects of other abused drugs which cause elevation of dopamine in the nucleus accumbens[34] needs to be considered.

MAO B inhibition by smoke may also reduce the levels of hydrogen peroxide, a by-product of MAO oxidation. The brain is particularly vulnerable to free radical oxidation and hydrogen peroxide production in excess of the detoxifying capacity of anti-oxidant enzymes has been postulated to lead to oxidative stress and neuro-degeneration.[36] MAO B inhibition resulting in decreased levels of hydrogen peroxide may be one of the mechanisms for the delay of the progression of Parkinson's disease with L-deprenyl treatment.[37]

Cigarette smoking poses a massive, yet potentially preventable, public health problem.[1,38] However, the development of more effective therapeutic strategies for treating that subgroup of individuals who consistently relapse after attempts to stop smoking requires a better understanding of the neuropsychopharmacological basis of why people smoke. This observation that cigarette smokers have a marked reduction in brain MAO B raises the possibility that other substances in addition to nicotine may contribute to the neuropharmacological properties of cigarette smoke and this variable needs to be considered in the behavioral and epidemiological characteristics of smoking and in treating smoking addiction. In fact, MAO A inhibitors have recently been reported to facilitate smoking cessation in highly dependent smokers.[39]

REFERENCES

1. Henningfield JE, Schuh LM, Jarvik ME. Pathophysiology of tobacco dependence. In: Bloom FE, Kupfer DJ, eds. Psychopharmacology, the Fourth Generation of Progress. Chapter 147. New York: Raven Press Ltd, 1995:1715-1729.

2. Jarvik ME, Schneider NG. In: Johnson JH, Ruiz R, Millman RB, Langood JG, eds. Substance-Abuse—A Comprehensive Textbook (2nd edition), Chapter 25 Baltimore: Williams and Wilkens, 1992:334-356.

3. Schelling TC. Addictive drugs: the cigarette experience. Science 1992; 255:430-433.

4. Baron JA. Cigarette smoking and Parkinson's disease. Neurology 1986; 36:1490-1496.

5. Morens DM, Grandinetti A, Reed D, White LR, Ross GW. Cigarette smoking and protection from Parkinson's disease: false association or etiological clue. Neurology 1995; 45:1041-1051.

6. Hughes JR, Hatsukama DK Mitchell JE, Dahlgren LA. Prevalence of smoking among psychiatric outpatients. Am J Psychiatry 1986; 143:993-997.

7. Glassman AH, Helzer JE, Covey LS, Cottler LB, Stetner F, Tipp JE, Johnson J. Smoking, smoking cessation, and major depression. JAMA 1990; 264: 1546-1549.

8. Henningfield JE, Clayton R, Pollen W. Involvement of tobacco in alcoholism and illictit drug use. Br J Addiction 1990; 85:279-292.

9. Singer T. Monoamine oxidases: old friends hold many surprises. FASEB J 1995; 9:605- 610.

10. Oreland L, Fowler CJ, Schalling D. Low platelet monoamine oxidase activity in cigarette smokers. Life Sci 1981; 29:2511-2518.

11. Norman TR, Chamberlain KG, French MA. Platelet monoamine oxidase: low activity in cigarette smokers. Psychiatry Res 1987; 20:199-205.

12. Yong VW, Perry TL. Monoamine oxidase B, smoking, and Parkinson's disease. J. Neurological Sci 1986; 72:265-272.

13. Berlin I, Saïd S, Spreux-Varoquaux O, Olivares R, Launay J-M, Puech AJ. Monoamine oxidase A and B activities in heavy smokers. Biol Psychiatry 1995; 38:756-761.

14. Yu PH, Boulton AA. Irreversible inhibition of MAO by some components of cigarette smoke. Life Sci 1987; 41:675.

15. Pavlin R, Sket D. Effect of cigarette smoke on brain monoamine oxidase activity. Farm vestn 1993; 44:185-192.

16. Carr LA, Basham JK. Effects of tobacco smoke constituents on MPTP-indiced toxicity and monoamine oxidase activity in the mouse brain. Life Sci 1991; 48:1173-1177.

17. Boulton AA, Yu PH, Tipton KF. Biogenic amine adducts, monoamine oxidase inhibitors, and smoking. Lancet 1988; 1:114-115.

18. Fowler JS, Wang G-J, Logan J, Xie S, Volkow ND, MacGregor RR, Schlyer DJ, Pappas N, Alexoff DL, Patlak C, Wolf AP. Selective reduction of radiotracer trapping by deuterium substitution: comparison of [^{11}C]L-deprenyl and [^{11}C]L-deprenyl-D2 for MAO B mapping. J Nucl Med. 1996; 36:1255- 1262.

19. Fowler JS, Wang G-J, Volkow ND, Pappas N, Logan J, MacGregor RR, Alexoff D, Wolf AP, Warner D, Cilento R, Zezulkova I. Inhibition of monoamine oxidase B in the brains of smokers. Nature 1996; 379:733-736.

20. Fowler JS, Wolf AP, MacGregor RR, Dewey SL, Logan J, Schlyer DJ, Langström B. Mechanistic PET studies: demonstration of a deuterium isotope effect in the MAO catalyzed binding of [^{11}C]L-deprenyl in living baboon brain. J Neurochem. 1988; 51:1524-1534.

21. Alexoff DL, Shea C, Wolf AP, Fowler JS, King P, Gatley SJ, Schlyer DJ. Plasma input function determination for PET using a commercial laboratory robot. Nucl. Med. Biol. 1995; 22:893-904.
22. Wang G-J, Volkow ND, Wolf AP, Brodie JD, Hitzemann R. Intersubject variability of brain glucose metabolic measurements in young normal males. J Nucl Med. 1994; 35:1457-1466.
23. Matsui T, Hirano A. An atlas of the human brain for computerized tomography. Stuttgart: Gustav Fischer, 1978.
24. Koeppe RA, Holthoff A, Frey KA, Kilbourn MR, Kuhl DE. Compartmental analysis of [^{11}C]flumazenil kinetics for the estimation of ligand transport rate and receptor distribution using positron emission tomography. J Cereb Blood Flow Metab. 1991; 11:735-744.
25. Logan J, Dewey SL, Wolf AP, Fowler JS, Brodie JD, Angrist B, Volkow ND, Gatley SJ. Effects of endogenous dopamine on measures of [^{18}F]N-methyl-spiroperidol binding in the basal ganglia: comparison of simulations and experimental results from PET studies in baboons. Synapse 1991; 9:195-207.
26. Fowler JS, Volkow ND, Logan J, Schlyer DJ, MacGregor RR, Wang G-J, Wolf AP, Pappas N, Alexoff D, Shea C, Dorflinger E, Yoo K, Morawsky L, Fazzini E. Monoamine oxidase B (MAO B) inhibitor therapy in Parkinson's disease: the degree and reversibility of human brain MAO B inhibition by Ro 19 6327 Neurology 1993; 43:1984-1992.
27. Patlak C, Fenstermacher JD, Blasberg RG. Graphical evaluation of blood-to-brain transfer constants from multiple time- activity data. J. Cereb. Blood Flow Metab. 1983; 3:1-7.
28. Blomqvist G. On the construction of functional maps in positron emission tomography. J. Cereb. Blood Flow Metab. 1984; 4:629-632.
29. Walpole RE, Myers RH. Tests of hypotheses. In: Probability and Statistics for Engineers and Scientists., 2nd edition, MacMillan Publishing Co. Inc. 1978: 256-259.
30. Yamashita K, Kobayashi S, Yamaguchi S, Kitani M, Tsunematsu T. Effect of smoking on regional cerebral blood flow in the normal aged volunteers. Gerontology 1988; 34:199-204.
31. Fowler JS, Volkow ND, Logan J, Wang G-J, MacGregor RR, Schlyer D, Wolf AP, Pappas N, Alexoff D, Shea C, Dorflinger E, Krochowy L, Yoo K, Fazzini E, Patlak C. Slow recovery of human brain MAO B after L-deprenyl (selegeline) withdrawal. Synapse 1994; 18: 86-93.
32. Glover V, Sandler M, Owen F, Riley GJ. Dopamine is a monoamine oxidase B substrate in man. Nature 1977; 265:80-81.
33. Di Chiara G, Imperato A. Drugs abused by humans preferentially increase synaptic dopamine concentrations in the mesolimbic system of freely moving rats. Proc Nat Acad USA. 1988; 85:5274-5278.
34. Pontieri FE, Tanda G, Orzi F, Di Chiera G. Effects of nicotine on the nucleus accumbens and similarity to those of addictive drugs. Nature. 1996; 382: 255-257.

35. McGeer PL, McGeer EG, Suzuki JS. Aging and extrapyramidal function. Arch Neurol 1977; 34:33-35.

36. Reiter RJ. Oxidative processes and antioxidative defense mechanisms in the aging brain. FASEB J. 1995; 9:526-533.

37. Tetrud JW, Langston JW. The effect of deprenyl (selegeline) on the natural history of Parkinson's disease. Science 1989; 245:519-522.

38. Benowitz NL. Pharmacologic aspects of cigarette smoking and nicotine addiction. New Eng J Med. 1988; 319:1318-1330.

39. Berlin I, Saïd S, Spreux-Varoquaux O, Launay J-M, Olivares R, Millet V, Lecrubier Y, Puech AJ. A reversible monoamine oxidase A inhibitor (moclobemide) facilitates smoking cessation and abstinence in heavy, dependent smokers. Clin Pharmac Ther 1995; 58:444-452.

Cigarette Smoking
and Major Depression

Lirio S. Covey, PhD
Alexander H. Glassman, MD
Fay Stetner, MA

SUMMARY. The authors review recent literature that has demonstrated an association between cigarette smoking behavior and major depression. Persons with major depression are more likely to smoke and to have difficulty when they try to stop. When they manage to succeed in stopping, such persons are at increased risk of experiencing mild to severe states of depression, including full blown major depression. The period of vulnerability to a new depressive episode appears to vary from a few weeks to several months after cessation. This knowledge suggests a relationship between smoking and depression that is complex, pernicious, and potentially life-long. It is recommended that cessation treatments incorporate screening procedures that will identify those patients with a propensity to depression and monitor the emergence of postcessation depression, particularly in those with a history of depression. *[Article copies available for a fee from The Haworth Document Delivery Service: 1-800-342-9678. E-mail address: getinfo@haworth.com]*

Lirio S. Covey, Alexander H. Glassman, and Fay Stetner are affiliated with the New York State Psychiatric Institute, Department of Psychiatry, College of Physicians and Surgeons, Columbia University, New York, NY.

Address correspondence to: Dr. Lirio S. Covey, PI 116, New York State Psychiatric Institute, 722 West 168th Street, New York, NY 10032.

[Haworth co-indexing entry note]: "Cigarette Smoking and Major Depression." Covey, Lirio S., Alexander H. Glassman, and Fay Stetner. Co-published simultaneously in *Journal of Addictive Diseases* (The Haworth Medical Press, an imprint of The Haworth Press, Inc.) Vol. 17, No. 1, 1998, pp. 35-46; and: *Smoking and Illicit Drug Use* (ed: Mark S. Gold, and Barry Stimmel) The Haworth Medical Press, an imprint of The Haworth Press, Inc., 1998, pp. 35-46. Single or multiple copies of this article are available for a fee from The Haworth Document Delivery Service [1-800-342-9678, 9:00 a.m. - 5:00 p.m. (EST). E-mail address: getinfo@haworth.com].

35

Research over the past several years has established an association between cigarette smoking and depression. Compared with nondepressed individuals, those with a vulnerability to depression are more likely to be smokers and to have difficulty when they attempt to stop. Additionally, the emergence of depressed mood and major depressive episodes following smoking cessation has been reported. In this paper, we review findings by our group and others that have illuminated various aspects of the link between major depression (MD) and smoking. These findings have been observed across several studies, with clinical and community-based samples, offering compelling evidence for a relationship between depression and smoking that is complex, pernicious, and potentially life-long.

MAJOR DEPRESSION AND SMOKING

In 1988, we reported a 60% prevalence rate of prior MD history in a placebo-controlled trial of clonidine for smoking cessation.[1] This was a striking observation since the figure is several times higher than the 10% average rate of MD that had been seen in community-based studies.[2] Since then, rates of past MD that range from 35% to 41% have been reported in other smoking cessation trials.[3-6] Although lower than our initial observation, those rates still indicate an overrepresention of depressed individuals among smokers seeking nicotine dependence treatment.

Epidemiological studies have also shown the frequent co-occurrence of cigarette smoking and major depression. In data from 3200 subjects seen in the St. Louis site of the National Institute of Mental Health-Epidemiological Catchment Area (NIMH-ECA) survey, the prevalence of lifetime major depression among those who had ever smoked cigarettes regularly was 10% compared with 6% in the general population.[7] In a sample of 1200 young adults enrolled in a health maintenance organization, Breslau found that the proportions of individuals who reported a lifetime history of major depression varied according to nicotine dependence/smoking status: 26.7% in nicotine dependent subjects, 12% in non-dependent smokers, and 9.4% in nonsmokers.[8] An elegant study of 1566 female twins by Kendler et al. not only found higher rates of major depression among smokers, it also suggested that a shared genetic factor explained the association.[9] In both latter studies, nicotine dependence[8] or number of cigarettes smoked[9] were directly associated with the prevalence of MD.

MAJOR DEPRESSION AND SMOKING CESSATION

That past MD impairs the ability to stop smoking was the second major observation in the clonidine trial cited earlier.[1] The very high rate of depression history among our subjects prompted us to examine the effect of such a history on cessation ability. We found that for both genders, but specially among women, past MD was a significant detriment to treatment success. Only 33% of the depressed subjects but 57% of the subjects without past MD had stopped smoking. The adverse influence of past MD was also observed in the cessation trials by Hall et al.[4,5] and Niaura et al.[6] and in epidemiological data from the NIMH-ECA survey in St. Louis.[7] In data collected from Durham, North Carolina, another site of the NIMH-ECA survey, the strongest effect on the ability to quit smoking was observed in the subgroup of females with a history of recurrent major depression.[10]

DEPRESSED MOOD DURING NICOTINE WITHDRAWAL

To understand how past MD affects smoking cessation outcome, we examined the withdrawal experience of smokers stratified by depression history. Our results showed that in addition to predicting failure, past MD affects the intensity of nicotine withdrawal as well.[11] Among 36 placebo-treated subjects in the earlier clinical study,[1] depressed mood and difficulty concentrating were experienced more frequently and more severely by smokers with past MD. Although the differences were not statistically significant, subjects with past MD also showed a tendency towards higher levels of craving, irritability, anxiety, and restlessness during the nicotine withdrawal period (Figure 1). Furthermore, both depressed mood and a global withdrawal symptom score predicted eventual treatment failure at the end of the four-week study period.[11] The propensity of smokers with past MD to experience depressed mood during nicotine withdrawal was also observed by Breslau et al.[12] and by Hughes.[13]

SEVERE DEPRESSION
WITHIN WEEKS OF SMOKING CESSATION

Prompted by encouraging results for clonidine from the first study, we began a second, larger trial of clonidine. We took this opportunity to investigate the effect of cessation on the occurrence of more serious depressive states. As we reported in a paper based on 300 participants,[3] severe depressions developed in eight subjects within a few weeks of stopping smoking. Six of these cases occurred among 113 subjects with a history of MD and one occurred among 34 subjects without that history but who had reported a history of alcoholism. The eighth case did not have

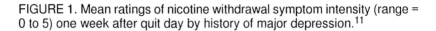

FIGURE 1. Mean ratings of nicotine withdrawal symptom intensity (range = 0 to 5) one week after quit day by history of major depression.[11]

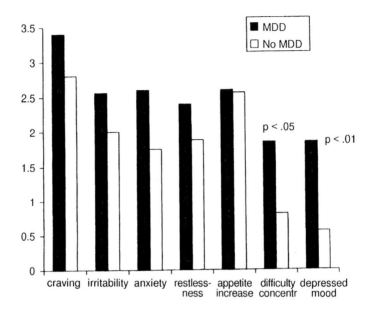

previous MD (nor alcoholism or dysthymia) but did report a suicidal attempt at age 13 and frequent bouts of depressed mood, none of which met the full DSM-IIIR criteria for MD.[14] All eight cases resumed smoking within days of experiencing the depression and quickly felt relief. Pertinent characteristics of these cases are shown in Table 1. It may be seen that our group of "depression casualties" were mostly female and that all had a psychiatric history (seven had past depression, one was a recovering alcoholic). However, there were wide dispersions in the subjects' age, their score on the Beck Depression Inventory (BDI)[15] taken at baseline, their level of nicotine dependence as measured by the Fagerstrom Tolerance Questionnaire (FTQ),[16] and the treatment medication they had received (4 out of 7 were on clonidine).

MAJOR DEPRESSION
AFTER SMOKING CESSATION TREATMENT

After the 10-week period of active treatment with medication (clonidine/placebo) and weekly individual behavior therapy, we followed up the

TABLE 1. Baseline characteristics of smokers who experienced depression while in smoking cessation treatment.

Patient #	Sex	Age	Psychiatric History	BDI[1]	FTQ[2]	Cigarettes smoked daily	Treatment
#1.	Male	32	Alcoholism	5	6	35	Clonidine
#2.	Female	44	Single MD[3]	1	4	20	Placebo
#3.	Female	68	Recurrent MD & Bipolar Disorder	0	9	50	Placebo
#4.	Male	36	Recurrent MD	2	8	40	Clonidine
#5.	Female	50	Single MD	12	6	30	Clonidine
#6.	Female	46	Depression[4]	12	8	45	Placebo
#7.	Female	24	Recurrent MD	5	7	25	Placebo
#8.	Female	62	Single MD	13	7	40	Clonidine
Means[5]	55% Female	45	20% Single MD 18% Recurrent MD 25% Alcoholism	5	6.8	32	51% Clonidine

1 Beck Depression Inventory
2 Fagerstrom Tolerance Questionnaire
3 Major Depression
4 Suicide attempt at age 13 and frequent bouts of depressed mood that did not meet DSM-IIIR criteria for major depression.
5 Data are based on the total sample of 300 participants who entered a placebo-controlled trial of clonidine.[3]

nicotine abstinent subjects over the course of 12 months. (Self-reports of abstinence at end-of-treatment were verified by serum cotinine level less than 15 ng/ml.) Since our a priori objective was to examine the incidence of long-term nicotine abstinence, we had decided at the outset of the study to follow up only those subjects who successfully stopped smoking. The absence of data from treatment failures limited our ability to examine the course of post-cessation events other than continued abstinence beyond the first three months of follow-up. Nevertheless, the three-month data yielded a strong, if not entirely surprising, finding. As reported elsewhere,[17] the proportion of new major depressive episodes was significantly greater among the abstinent subjects who had a history of either recurrent or single MD compared with subjects without that history (30%, 16%, 2%, respectively, p < 0.001) (Figure 2). This effect remained statistically significant (p < 0.01) after controlling for possible confounding due to age, gender, baseline Fagerstrom score, depressed mood at baseline, depressed mood at end-of-treatment, and withdrawal symptom score at end-of-treatment. Further analysis showed that other variables including number of cigarettes smoked at baseline, the type (i.e., nicotine yield) of the cigarette smoked, duration of smoking history, prior medical conditions, and use of other drugs were unrelated to the onset of new depressive episodes.

Pertinent details of these post-treatment cases of major depression are shown in Table 2. Like the group who became depressed within weeks of

FIGURE 2. Incidence of major depression three months after completing smoking cessation treatment by history of major depression.[17]

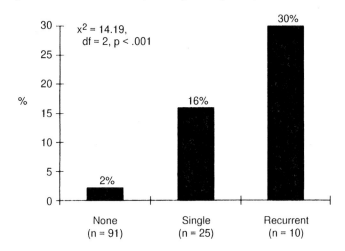

TABLE 2. Baseline, end-of-treatment, and Month 3 characteristics of subjects who became depressed within 3 months of ending a 10-week smoking cessation treatment. All were nicotine abstinent at Week 10, verified by serum cotinine <15 ng/ml.

Patient #	Sex	Age	Baseline				End-of-treatment			Month 3
			Psychiatric History	BDI[1]	FTQ[2]	Cigarettes smoked daily	Treatment	BDI	Withdrawal Symptom Score	Cigarettes smoked daily
#1.	F	33	Single MD[3]	6	8	30	Placebo	1	11	0
#2.	F	44	Recurrent MD & Panic Disorder	2	7	70	Clonidine	7	13	0
#3.	F	55	Single MD	5	6	20	Clonidine	9	17	1
#4.	M	37	Single MD	20	7	55	Placebo	29	24	35
#5.	F	49	Recurrent MD	1	8	50	Clonidine	0	8	50
#6.	F	42	No history	1	7	35	Placebo	22	31	0
#7.	F	46	No history	7	7	20	Placebo	3	19	0
#8.	F	42	Recurrent MD	0	5	20	Clonidine	11	16	0
#9.	M	35	Single MD	3	5	40	Placebo	10	9	0
Means[4]	F = 50%	46	72% No MD 20% Single MD 8% Recurrent MD	4	6.5	30	54% Clonidine	3.5	8.2	64% = 0 cpd

[1] Beck Depression Inventory
[2] Fagerstrom Tolerance Questionnaire
[3] Major Depression
[4] Data are based on 126 treatment successes at Week 10 and reached at Month 3 follow-up.

nicotine abstinence (Table 1), subjects who became depressed more than 10 weeks after they had stopped smoking were also likely to be female (7/9) and to have a history of major depression (7/9). All but one received an FTQ score greater than 7, indicating high dependence. Although all but one rated beyond the group mean for all successful abstainers on the global withdrawal symptom measure at Week 10, there was no consistent effect of depressed mood at baseline or at end of treatment. These nine subjects were neither among our youngest or our oldest subjects (age range was 33 to 55 years) and whether the treatment received was cloni-dine or placebo was not a factor. Interestingly, stressful life events during the last four weeks of the 10-week treatment period were reported by the only two subjects without a prior psychiatric history. Patient #6's son-in-law who was working overseas had been hospitalized, her daughter had left to be with the husband, and her grandson had come to live with her for the duration of her daughter's absence. Patient #7 reported that both her father and her father-in-law had become seriously ill, and she would be making a trip out-of-state to be with her father.

Of further interest, six had remained nicotine abstinent when reached at Month 3. Five of them had been treated with an antidepressant medication. One case who chose to "tough it out" and not use antidepressant medica-tion was no longer depressed and still not smoking when seen at her sixth month follow-up visit. One subject had begun to smoke one cigarette daily (she was smoking at her pre-treatment level of 20 cigarettes a day when seen three months later). Patient #4 resumed smoking despite treatment with an antidepressant. By the time we reached her at Month 3, Patient #5's depression had resolved, but she was smoking at her baseline level of 50 cigarettes daily.

It may be argued that the absence of information from a control group of treatment failures does not allow us to conclude that cessation provoked the onset of new depressive episodes. It is true that individuals who have been depressed are more likely to experience depression in the future. Nevertheless, we wish to point out that the 20% recurrence rate during a rather brief period (three months) among the 35 cases with previous MD is unusually high, particularly in view of the fact that all had been free of the diagnosis for at least six months before beginning the smoking cessation treatment. For perspective, it is noted that the rate of MD after cessation in this group is similar to the recurrence rate reported in a relapse study of currently depressed individuals who had been treated for major depres-sion.[18] In the case of patients #6 and #7, both of whom did not have a psychiatric history, one could speculate, as might be posited by Brown and Harris,[19] that the stressful life events that they experienced contributed to the depressive episode. Perhaps neurophysiological alterations involved in nicotine withdrawal[20] or simply the loss of smoking as a coping tool diminished their customary ability to withstand a stressful life event.

To summarize, data obtained from participants in two clinical trials suggest that the risk of post-cessation depression, though small among smokers who do not have a psychiatric history, is considerable among those with a history of MD. The affected cases were predominantly women, but as suggested by a regression analysis which found no effect of gender,[17] the higher frequency of major depression history among women may account for that observation.

CLINICAL IMPLICATIONS

A clinical implication of these findings is the importance of ascertaining at screening the patient's vulnerability to depression. At a minimum, this can be accomplished by probing if the patient has ever experienced depressed mood nearly every day for an extended period of two weeks or more. A positive reply would merit further questions related to the co-occurrence of loss of pleasure and physical signs such as marked disturbances in sleep, appetite, ability to concentrate and energy level. Alternatively, the smoking cessation clinician could administer any one of a number of measurements that tap current feelings of depression such as the Beck Depression Inventory (BDI) and the Center for Epidemiologic Studies Depression Scale (CES-D). Although such symptom inventories are not diagnostic of major depression, elevated scores (a BDI greater than 10 and a CES-D greater than 16) are useful indicators of a possible propensity to depressive illness. While all smokers who quit need to be monitored, patients who test positively on such procedures for screening depression require closer supervision.

RESEARCH IMPLICATIONS

Further work is needed to ascertain the determinants of major depression following smoking cessation, the latency of its onset, and its effect on the resumption of smoking. It is noteworthy that although depressed mood or severe depression occurring immediately after cessation appeared to decrease the likelihood of sustaining abstinence,[3,10] severe depression occurring several weeks after quitting did not exact an immediate return to smoking.

Knowledge about the link between depression and smoking has influenced recent efforts to develop pharmacological and psychological smoking cessation interventions. These efforts are important since those who continue to smoke in spite of widespread prohibitions against smoking are likely to be the ones who are most addicted or who also suffer from a psychiatric or psychological problem. Positive results from clinical trials of antidepressants, i.e., doxepin,[21] bupropion[22] and nortriptyline[23] as cessation aids with broad groups of smokers suggest the utility of these medications for smokers with past MD. Our own clinical work has seen similar positive outcomes with bupropion and nortriptyline, and among smokers with past MD, with fluoxetine and sertraline. Negative results from a large trial of fluoxetine for smoking cessation that involved smokers irrespective of major depression (psychiatric history was not ascertained) have been reported.[24] The seemingly contradictory findings about fluoxetine, a serotonin reuptake inhibitor, may indicate specificity in nicotine-receptor regulation among different classes of antidepressants, implying that different classes of antidepressants will vary in their effects for different types of smokers. Controlled trials to address this important issue are needed.

The usefulness of nicotine replacement therapy for smokers with a propensity to depression also requires investigation. Bock et al. have reported one case where the nicotine patch reversed a developing post-cessation depression.[25] Indeed, one could expect that nicotine replacement would reduce the risk of post-cessation major depression.[26] However, we have also observed the emergence of severe depression requiring treatment in two female patients who stopped smoking while using 21 mg transdermal nicotine. This would indicate the need for additional intervention for certain smokers with a greater vulnerability to depression.

The general consensus in smoking cessation treatment and research is that concomitant behavior therapy improves the outcome of pharmacological treatments. The content and form (duration, frequency, group or individual) of psychological counseling that will be most helpful and most cost-effective for smokers with comorbid depression is largely unknown. Our own clinical experience suggests the usefulness of counseling techniques that are directive yet encouraging of emotional expression for the smoker with past MD. Moreover, the literature offers some clues. Hall et al. found that, among smokers with past MD, the cessation rate was higher among those who received behavior therapy oriented towards mood management than among those who received a health eduction behavior counseling.[4,27] A study by Zelman et al. found that supportive counseling was more helpful than a skills training approach for smokers with high negative affect.[28]

Other questions relevant to nicotine dependence treatment of smokers with depression need further investigation. A relapse study of patients who were treated for major depression found that the risk of a recurrent episode declines over time.[18] Will the risk of depression after smoking cessation follow a similar pattern? When there is comorbidity, for example, from alcoholism or anxiety, will smoking cessation provoke or exacerbate the comorbid condition as well? Finally, what conditions or treatments can avert the potential negative consequences of smoking cessation? While there has been abundant work and information about the physical consequences of smoking and smoking cessation, research efforts regarding psychiatric aspects are clearly just beginning.

REFERENCES

1. Glassman AH, Stetner F, Walsh BT, Raizman PS, Fleiss JL, Cooper TB, Covey LS. Heavy smokers, smoking cessation, and clonidine: Results of a double-blind, randomized trial. JAMA 1988;259:2863-2866.

2. Baldessarini RJ. Risk rates for depression. Arch Gen Psychiatry 1984; 41:103-104.

3. Glassman AH, Covey LS, Dalack GW, Stetner F, Rivelli SK, Fleiss JL, Cooper TB. Smoking cessation, clonidine, and vulnerability to nicotine among dependent smokers. Clin Pharmacol Ther 1993;54:670-679.

4. Ginsberg D, Hall SM, Reus VI, Munoz RF. Mood and depression diagnosis in smoking cessation. Experimental and Clinical Psychopharmacology 1995; 3:389-395.

5. Hall SM, Munoz RF, Reus VI. Cognitive-behavioral intervention increases abstinence rates for depressive-history smokers. J Consult Clin Psychol 1994; 62:141-146.

6. Niaura R, Goldstein MG, Depue J, Keuthen N, Kristeller J, Abrams D. Fluoxetine, symptoms of depression, and smoking cessation (abstract). Annals of Behavioral Medicine 1995;17, Suppl:S061.

7. Glassman AH, Helzer JE, Covey LS, Cottler LB, Stetner F, Tipp JE, Johnson J. Smoking, smoking cessation, and major depression. JAMA 1990;264: 1546-1549.

8. Breslau N. Psychiatric comorbidity of smoking and nicotine dependence. Behav Genet 1995;25:95-101.

9. Kendler KS, Neale MC, MacLean CJ, Heath AC, Eaves LJ, Kessler RC. Smoking and major depression: A causal analysis. Arch Gen Psychiatry 1993; 50:36-43.

10. Covey LS, Hughes DC, Glassman AH, Blazer DG, George LK. Eversmoking, quitting, and psychiatric disorders: evidence from the Durham, North Carolina, Epidemiologic Catchment Area. Tobacco Control 1994;3:222-227.

11. Covey LS, Glassman AH, Stetner F. Depression and depressive symptoms in smoking cessation. Compr Psychiatry 1990;31:350-354.

12. Breslau N, Kilbey MM, Andreski P. Nicotine withdrawal symptoms and psychiatric disorders: Findings from an epidemiologic study of young adults. Am J Psychiatry 1992;149:464-469.

13. Hughes JR. Tobacco withdrawal in self-quitters. J Consult Clin Psychol 1992;60:689-697.

14. American Psychiatric Association. Diagnostic and Statistical Manual of Mental Disorders, Third Edition, Revised. Washington DC: Amercian Psychiatric Association, 1987.

15. Beck AT, Ward CH, Mendelson M, Mock J, Erbaugh J. An inventory for measuring depression. Arch Gen Psychiatry 1961;4:561-571.

16. Fagerstrom KO. Measuring degree of physical dependence to tobacco smoking with reference to individualization of treatment. Addict Behav 1978; 3:235-241.

17. Covey LS, Glassman AH, Stetner F. Major depression following smoking cessation. Am J Psychiatry 1997;154:263-265.

18. Keller MB, Lavori PW, Lewis CE, Klerman GL. Predictors of relapse in major depressive disorder. JAMA 1983;250:3299-3304.

19. Brown GW, Harris T. Social Origins of Depression. New York: Free Press, 1978.

20. Carmody TP. Affect regulation, nicotine addiction, and smoking cessation. J Psychoactive Drugs 1989;21:331-342.

21. Edwards NB, Simmons RC, Rosenthal TL, Hoon PW, Downs JM. Doxepin in the treatment of nicotine withdrawal. Psychosomatics 1988;29:203-206.

22. Ferry LH, Robbins AS, Scariati PD, Masterson A, Abbey DE, Burchette RJ. Enhancement of smoking cessation using the antidepressant, bupropion hydrochloride. Circulation 1992;86(4):I-671.(Abstract)

23. Hall SM. New directions in medications for the treatment of tobacco dependence. Washington, DC, March 15-17, 1996: Presented at the Society for Research on Nicotine and Tobacco, 2nd Annual Conference.

24. Mizes JS, Sloan DM, Segraves K, Spring B, Pingatore R, Kristeller J. Fluoxetine and weight gain in smoking cessation: Examination of actual weight gain and fear of weight gain. Boca Raton, FL. Presented at The New Clinical Drug Evaluation Unit Program, 36th Annual Meeting, May 28-31, 1996.

25. Bock BC, Goldstein MG, Marcus BH. Depression following smoking cessation in women. J Subst Abuse 1996;8:137-144.

26. Foulds J. A role for dopamine in nicotine psychosis? Addiction 1991; 91: 1388-1389.

27. Hall SM, Munoz RF, Reus VI. Depression and smoking treatment: A clinical trial of an affect regulation treatment. NIDA Res Monogr 1992;119:326.

28. Zelman DC, Brandon TH, Jorenby DE, Baker TB. Measures of affect and nicotine dependence predict differential response to smoking cessation treatments. J Consult Clin Psychol 1992;60:943-952.

Caffeine and Nicotine Use in an Addicted Population

Lon R. Hays, MD
David Farabee, PhD
Will Miller, PA

SUMMARY. This study was undertaken to examine differences in caffeine and nicotine use between the psychiatric population and the addicted population in a private psychiatric inpatient facility. Eighty-six patients on an adult addictive disease inpatient unit and 80 patients on an adult psychiatry unit in a private psychiatric hospital were interviewed with regard to their use of nicotine and caffeine. In addition, demographic information and primary diagnoses were obtained from the psychiatric admission assessment in the medical record as listed by the admitting psychiatrist. Although there was little difference in psychiatric patients vs. chemically dependent patients with regard to the percentage of caffeine users, the chemically dependent individuals drank more coffee, soft drinks, and tea. A much greater percentage of the chemically dependent individuals also smoked cigarettes, although not in a greater amount than the psychiatric patients who smoked. Because group assignment was not random, ordinary least squares (OLS) regression analyses were conducted to determine the independent associations of age, sex, educa-

Lon R. Hays, David Farabee, and Will Miller are affiliated with the Department of Psychiatry, University of Kentucky Medical Center, Lexington, KY.

Address correspondence to: Lon R. Hays, University of Kentucky College of Medicine, Department of Psychiatry, Kentucky Clinic, Wing B, Lexington, KY 40536-0284.

[Haworth co-indexing entry note]: "Caffeine and Nicotine Use in an Addicted Population." Hays, Lon R., David Farabee, and Will Miller. Co-published simultaneously in *Journal of Addictive Diseases* (The Haworth Medical Press, an imprint of The Haworth Press, Inc.) Vol. 17, No. 1, 1998, pp. 47-54; and: *Smoking and Illicit Drug Use* (ed: Mark S. Gold, and Barry Stimmel) The Haworth Medical Press, an imprint of The Haworth Press, Inc., 1998, pp. 47-54. Single or multiple copies of this article are available for a fee from The Haworth Document Delivery Service [1-800-342-9678, 9:00 a.m. - 5:00 p.m. (EST). E-mail address: getinfo@haworth.com].

tion, and treatment population in predicting levels of caffeine and tobacco use. Even after controlling for demographic differences between the two samples, chemically dependent patients still reported higher levels of daily caffeine and tobacco use than patients on the general psychiatric unit. *[Article copies available for a fee from The Haworth Document Delivery Service: 1-800-342-9678. E-mail address: getinfo@haworth.com]*

INTRODUCTION

There is a growing body of literature regarding caffeine and nicotine use, although the use of these substances among psychiatric patients and addicted individuals needs more study. DSM-IV identifies caffeine as one of the eleven classes of substances (DSM-IV)[1] although it's not considered to cause abuse or dependence.[2] In spite of this, there are well-known signs of caffeine intoxication including pupillary dilation, diaphoresis, restlessness, nervousness, excitement, flushed face, muscle twitching, psychomotor agitation, and pressured speech.[2]

Many studies have examined the physiological and psychological effects of caffeine; although evidence is often contradictory, numerous psychiatric units control or limit caffeinated products.[3] A higher incidence of psychosis and higher levels of state anxiety as well as higher scores on the Beck Depression Inventory has been found in heavy caffeine users. Less anxiety, irritability, and hostility has been seen when decaffeinated coffee was substituted for caffeinated coffee on a ward of long-stay psychiatric patients. On the other hand, decaffeinated coffee has not been found to improve the behavior of 33 schizophrenic inpatients and no correlation has been found between caffeine consumption and levels of anxiety and depression in a study of long-stay schizophrenic patients. A tendency for caffeine consumption to decrease with age and for men to consume more caffeine than women was observed. There was no correlation with cigarette smoking. Others have reported that cigarette smoking and caffeine intake correlate in normal subjects as well as in psychiatric patients.[4]

Goff et al. reported that the number of cigarettes smoked daily was positively correlated with the daily intake of caffeine in a group of schizophrenic outpatients. Caffeine use was associated with elevation of psychosis, but there was little evidence to suggest that it directly worsened their clinical state.[4]

Although little is written about the prevalence of caffeine use among psychiatric patients, the prevalence of cigarette use is between 35 and 54 percent, compared to 30 to 35 percent in the general population.[5] The rate of smoking among patients admitted for substance use disorders is 75 to 90 percent.[6] Smoking is the most modifiable risk factor for cardiovascular and pulmonary disease; and tobacco and alcohol act in synergy to increase the risk of esophageal cancer, head and neck cancers and hypertension.[6] In spite of this, most treatment programs treat nicotine as a less serious problem than other drugs and alcohol. Possible reasons for this include: (1) fear that smoking cessation would be stressful for this population, (2) the belief that smoking is a less important problem that other forms of drug use, (3) staff smoking practices, and (4) fear that programs might lose clients if they include treatment for nicotine dependence.[6]

Some studies have shown that abstention from alcohol and smoking are highly correlated. One study of veterans in a substance abuse treatment program showed that most were interested in quitting smoking, believed that inpatient treatment was the best time to quit, and that quitting would not threaten their sobriety.[7]

In the late 1980's, bans on smoking became more prevalent and the first reports of limiting smoking on inpatient psychiatric units emerged. Psychiatric units were often exempt from no-smoking requirement; but that ended in 1992 when the Joint Commission on Accreditation of Healthcare Organizations required facilities to enforce "a hospital wide smoking policy that prohibits the use of smoking materials throughout the hospital.[8] There were numerous concerns that forced smoking cessation would cause patient distress, agitation, early discharges, or even violence.[9] Some studies have focused on the increased smoking rates in schizophrenia (over 80%),[5] and the belief that smoking produces relaxation or decreased anxiety in these patients as well as reducing medication side effects.

Various studies have examined the effect of smoking bans on psychiatric units. Velasco et al. found no major behavioral disruption occurred and there were no increases in use of restraints or seclusion or in discharges against medical advice. More verbal assaults and prescribing of prn medications for anxiety occurred immediately after the ban (but not in their comparison two years later).[10] Taylor et al., in a prospective study, found no significant difference between pre-ban and post-ban unit disruption and also found a shift in staff being in favor of the ban.[9] Resnick and Bosworth surveyed patient and staff attitudes before the ban and after its initiation and found staff approval increased from 24% to 95%.[11]

Many of the above mentioned studies have examined either the psychiatric population or the addicted population in a state hospital or VA facility. This study was undertaken to examine differences in caffeine and nicotine use between the psychiatric population and the addicted population in a private psychiatric inpatient facility.

METHODS

Eighty-six patients on an adult addictive disease inpatient unit and 80 patients on an adult psychiatry unit in a private psychiatric hospital were interviewed with regard to their use of nicotine and caffeine. Specific questions asked included:

1. Do you drink caffeinated coffee?
2. Do you drink caffeinated soft drinks?
3. Do you drink caffeinated tea?
4. Do you smoke cigarettes?
5. Do you chew tobacco?
6. Do you use snuff?

The 166 patients were interviewed over a four-month time period and were asked to quantify their daily use of each substance. Demographic information obtained included age, sex, race, and educational level. Primary diagnosis was obtained from the psychiatric admission assessment in the medical record as listed by the admitting psychiatrist. Patients with a primary diagnosis of a substance use disorder and another Axis I disorder were omitted from the survey.

RESULTS

Mean age of patients on the two units was similar (psychiatric inpatients-39.9; chemically dependent inpatients-41.2); however, there were 46 females on the psychiatric unit compared to 17 on the chemical dependence unit. Mean educational level of the two groups was 12.6 years. A large percentage of both populations were caffeine users: 91.3% of the psychiatric patients and 92.5% of the chemically dependent patients. A larger percentage of the chemically dependent patients were coffee drinkers (68.8% vs. 57.5%) and they drank an average of 5.5 cups/day compared to 3.4 cups/day. A larger percentage of the chemically dependent patients drank soft drinks (68.8% vs. 63.8%) and drank 4.5 soft drinks/day vs. 4.2/day for the psychiatric patients. A similar percentage of the two populations drank tea, but once again the chemically dependent group consumed more: 2.7 glasses/day vs. 1.7/day. In terms of nicotine use, 83.8% of the chemically dependent individuals used nicotine (81.2% smoked cigarettes) and 57.5% of the psychiatric patients used nicotine (53.8% smoked cigarettes). Among smokers, both populations smoked an average of 1.5 packs/day. The primary diagnosis on the adult psychiatric service was major depression (68.8% of patients) and on the chemical dependence unit, alcohol dependence (71.3% of patients) (see Table 1).

Because assignment to one of these two treatment populations was not random, it was possible that some of the variation in caffeine and tobacco use could be attributed to other demographic differences between patients on the addictive unit and the general population of psychiatric inpatients. To control for these possible effects, ordinary least squares (OLS) regression analyses were conducted to determine the independent associations of age, sex, education, and treatment population in predicting levels of caffeine and tobacco use. As shown in Table 2, age was the only demographic variable that was significantly associated with levels of daily caffeine consumption, with younger patients reporting higher levels of use. In addition, treatment condition also remained a significant predictor in the equation, with chemically dependent patients reporting higher levels of caffeine use, even after controlling for the effects of these other variables. Likewise, Table 3 presents the results of this same regression model predicting the number of cigarettes smoked daily. Higher rates of tobacco use were associated with being male, having fewer years of education, and being a patient on the chemical dependency unit.

DISCUSSION

In this population from a private psychiatric facility, there was little difference in psychiatric patients vs. chemically dependent patients with regard to the percentage of caffeine users; however, the chemically dependent individuals drank more coffee, soft drinks, and tea. A much greater percentage of the chemically dependent individuals smoked cigarettes, although not in a greater amount than the psychiatric patients who smoked. The percentage of psychiatric patients in this study who smoked was greater than the range generally quoted in other studies.[7] This is remarkable since there were very few schizophrenics who generally have the highest smoking rate among psychiatric patients.

There is certainly a debate as to whether smoking cessation may improve the chances of maintaining sobriety, but studies have shown that nicotine dependence treatment can be delivered without a deleterious effect on desired drug and alcohol treatment outcomes.[12,6] The high rate of

TABLE 1. Sample Characteristics

	PSYCHIATRIC INPATIENTS	CHEMICALLY DEPENDENT INPTS
	N = 80	N = 86
Mean Age	39.9	41.2
Age Range	18-79	18-75
Sex:		
Male	42.5%	79.1%
Female	57.5%	20.9%
Race:		
Caucasian	100%	97.7%
African-Amer.	0%	2.3%
Mean Ed. Level	12.5	12.7
Caffeine Users	73 (91.3%)	80 (93%)
Coffee	46 (3.4 cups/day)	59 (5.5 cups/day)**
Soft Drinks	51 (4.3 s.d./day)	60 (4.4 s.d./day)
Tea	24 (1.7/day)	27 (2.6/day)
Nicotine Users	46 (57.5%)	69 (80.2%)**
Cigarettes	43 (53.8%)	69 (80.2%)**
Avg.	1.5 packs/day	1.6 packs/day
Chewers	5	1
Snuff Users	1	2
Diagnoses:		
Maj. Depression	55	Alcohol Dep. 59
B.A.D.	9	Opioid Dep. 15
Psychosis	5	Cocaine Dep. 7
PTSD	4	Cannabis Dep. 5
Panic Disorder	3	Benzo. Dep. 5
Anorexia	2	

**$p < .01$

cigarette smoking among the addicted population in our study certainly supports the notion that there is tremendous need for smoking cessation as an integral part of an addictive disease program. The literature stresses the need for staff to accept nicotine as a drug of dependence, which is sometimes difficult, because of the chronic, rather than acute, nature of the

TABLE 2. Regression Model Predicting Level of Caffeine Consumption (Cups/Glasses Consumed per Day)

Variable	Parameter Estimate	Prob.
Intercept	10.5	.0001
Age	−.08	.005
Sex*	1.1	.23
Education	−.19	.14
Treatment Population**	2.2	.01

* 0 = Female, 1 = Male
** 0 = General Psychiatric Unit, 1 = Chemical Dependency Unit

Model: $F_{(4, 165)} = 5.6$, $R^2 = .12$, $p < .0003$

TABLE 3. Regression Model Predicting Number of Cigarettes Smoked per Day

Variable	Parameter Estimate	Prob.
Intercept	7.5	.0001
Age	−.23	.02
Sex*	2.2	.49
Education	−1.4	.003
Treatment Population**	8.5	.007

* 0 = Female, 1 = Male
** 0 = General Psychiatric Unit, 1 = Chemical Dependency Unit

Model: $F_{(4, 154)} = 6.1$, $R^2 = .13$, $p < .0001$

problems it causes. One of the limitations of the current study is that attitudes toward smoking cessation were not examined; others have reported that up to one third of patients in treatment desire simultaneous treatment for all of their addictive disorders including nicotine dependence.[12]

Several factors seem to support the notion of treating nicotine dependence in treatment facilities: (1) There's more widespread emphasis on overall health maintenance while smoking-induced deaths account for 15% of all mortality in the United States.[12] (2) Third party payors are more supportive of wellness and preventive measures. (3) There continue to be advances in nicotine-replacement therapy. As Joseph et al. pointed out, treatment for other drugs may provide "a teachable moment" and a unique opportunity to educate patients about the risk of smoking and use of cessation methods.[6]

If the challenge of improving the health of our overall population is to be met, our psychiatric patients and addicted patients must be included, if not targeted for smoking cessation programs.

REFERENCES

1. American Psychiatric Association: Diagnostic and Statistical Manual of Mental Disorders, Fourth Edition. Washington, DC, American Psychiatric Press 1994.

2. Schottenfeld RS, Assessment of the patient. In The American Psychiatric Press Textbook of Substance Abuse Treatment. Eds. M. Galanter and HD. Kleber, American Psychiatric Press, Inc., Washington, DC, 1994; pp.26-29.

3. Mayo KM, Falkowski W, Jones CAH, Caffeine use and effects in long-term psychiatric patients. British J of Psychiatry, 1993; 162: 543-545.

4. Goff DC, Henderson DC, Amico E, Cigarette smoking in schizophrenia: relationship to psychopathology and medication side effects. Am J Psychiatry 1992; 149:1189-1194.

5. DeLeon J, Dadvand M, Canuso C, White AO, Stanilla JK, Simpson GM, Schizophrenia and smoking: an epidemiological survey in a state hospital. Am J Psychiatry 1995;152:453-455.

6. Joseph AM, Nichol KL, Effect of treatment for nicotine dependence on alcohol and drug treatment outcomes, Addictive Behaviors 1993; 18: 635-644.

7. Irving LM, Seidner AL, Burling TA, Thomas RG, Brenner GF, Drug and alcohol abuse inpatients' attitudes about smoking cessation. J Subs Abuse 1994;6:267-278.

8. Appelbaum PS, Do hospitalized psychiatric patients have a right to smoke? Psych Services 1995;46(7):653-660.

9. Taylor NE, Rosenthal RN, Chabus B, Levine S, Hoffman AS, Reynolds J, Santos L, Willets I, Friedman P, The feasibility of smoking bans on psychiatric units. Gen Hosp Psych 1993;15:36-40.

10. Velasco J, Eells TD, Anderson R, Head M, Ryabik B, Mount R, Lippman S, A two-year follow-up on the effects of a smoking ban in an inpatient psychiatric service. Psych Services 1996;47(8):869-871.

11. Resnick MP, Bosworth EE, A smokefree psych unit. Hosp Comm Psych 1989; 40:525-529.

12. Hurt RD, Eberman KM, Croghan IT, Offord KD, Davis LJ, Morse RM, Palmen MA, Bruce BK, Nicotine dependence treatment during inpatient treatment for other additions: a prospective intervention trial. Alcohol Clin Exp Res 1994;18(40:867-872.

13. Hughes JR, An overview of nicotine use disorders for alcohol/drug abuse clinicians. The Am J. on Addictions 1996;5:262-274.

Comorbid Cigarette and Alcohol Addiction: Epidemiology and Treatment

Norman S. Miller, MD
Mark S. Gold, MD

SUMMARY. The close association of nicotine addiction and alcoholism is well established. As many as 80% of alcoholics smoke, and 30% of smokers are alcoholics. The mortality from cigarette smoking and alcoholism individually is very high, as an estimated 400,000 deaths from tobacco and 100,000 deaths from alcoholism are reported annually. Cigarettes and alcohol interact to cause certain cancers, e.g., head and neck. Only recently has attention been focused on the role of tobacco in abstinent alcoholics. An important study found high rates of mortality from tobacco in abstinent alcoholics in recovery. However, the mortality rates from alcoholism were high and predominant. Of great importance is that studies show that abstinence from alcohol essentially eliminates the premature deaths or increased mortality rates from active alcoholism. Similar studies showing a reduction in mortality from abstinence in nicotine addiction have not been forthcoming. The importance of treating nicotine addiction, however, is clear to reduce the high mortality rates from tobacco smoking in active or abstinent alcoholics. *[Article copies available for a fee from The Haworth Document Delivery Service: 1-800-342-9678. E-mail address: getinfo@haworth.com]*

Norman S. Miller is Chief, Division of Addictions Programs, and Associate Professor of Psychiatry and Neurology, Department of Psychiatry, University of Illinois at Chicago, Chicago, IL.

Mark S. Gold is Professor, Departments of Neuroscience, Psychiatry, Community Health & Family Medicine, University of Florida Brain Institute, Gainesville, FL.

Address correspondence to: Norman S. Miller, University of Illinois at Chicago, Department of Psychiatry, 912 South Wood Street, Chicago, IL 60612.

[Haworth co-indexing entry note]: "Comorbid Cigarette and Alcohol Addiction: Epidemiology and Treatment." Miller, Norman S., and Mark S. Gold. Co-published simultaneously in *Journal of Addictive Diseases* (The Haworth Medical Press, an imprint of The Haworth Press, Inc.) Vol. 17, No. 1, 1998, pp. 55-66; and: *Smoking and Illicit Drug Use* (ed: Mark S. Gold, and Barry Stimmel) The Haworth Medical Press, an imprint of The Haworth Press, Inc., 1998, pp. 55-66. Single or multiple copies of this article are available for a fee from The Haworth Document Delivery Service [1-800-342-9678, 9:00 a.m. - 5:00 p.m. (EST). E-mail address: getinfo@haworth.com].

55

EPIDEMIOLOGY OF TOBACCO AND ALCOHOL

That nicotine and alcohol addictions are chronic, fatal diseases is known from clinical experience and diverse studies. As an example, a recent survey of the actual causes of death in the United States between 1977 and 1993 categorized deaths according to the following "external (nongenetic) factors": tobacco (estimated 400,000 deaths), diet and activity patterns (300,000), alcohol (100,000), microbial agents (90,000), toxic agents (60,000), firearms (35,000), sexual behavior (30,000), motor vehicles (25,000), and illicit drug use (20,000) (Table 1). The study overlooked the known genetic contributions of addictive illnesses, namely, nicotine addiction and alcoholism, by attributing these conditions to roles of external factors.[1]

As an illustration, in 1990 the number of deaths due to other causes, largely genetic, and external factors, were heart disease (720,000), cancer (505,000), cerebrovascular disease (144,000), accidents (92,000), chronic obstructive pulmonary disease (87,000), pneumonia and influenza (80,000)

TABLE 1. Actual Causes of Death in the United States in 1990 (Reprinted from JAMA 270(18):2207-2212, 1993)

Cause	Estimated Number*	% of Total Deaths
Tobacco	400,000	19
Diet/activity patterns	300,000	14
Alcohol	100,000	5
Microbial agents	90,000	4
Toxic agents	60,000	3
Firearms	35,000	2
Sexual behavior	30,000	1
Motor vehicles	25,000	1
Illicit use of drugs	20,000	< 1
Total	1,060,000	50

*Composite approximation drawn from studies that use different approaches to derive estimates, ranging from actual counts (e.g., firearms) to population attributable risk calculations (e.g., tobacco). Numbers over 100,000 rounded to the nearest 100,000; over 50,000, rounded to the nearest 10,000; below 50,000, rounded to the nearest 5,000.

diabetes mellitus (48,000), suicide (31,000), chronic liver disease and cirrhosis (26,000), and human immunodeficiency virus (HIV) infection (25,000).[2] The authors did not view these conditions as analogous to addictive illness by including nicotine and alcoholism as diseases.[3] However, the comparison of coronary artery disease and cancer with nicotine addiction and alcoholism show compelling similarities among these conditions. Genetic influences in addictive disease (tobacco), coronary artery disease, cancer, and lifestyle behaviors are associated with all the conditions. Also, early detection and treatment can significantly alter the course of each set of these chronic diseases. Moreover, the contribution of tobacco addiction to deaths in these conditions has been established.[3]

The influence of certain conditions such as continued tobacco use with successful treatment of other associated conditions, such as abstinence from alcohol in alcoholism was only recently documented. The importance of treating all contributing external and genetic influences is illustrated by increased mortality from continued tobacco use in abstinent alcoholics.[4]

MORTALITY FROM TOBACCO

The contributions of tobacco to mortality are estimated to cause: 11 to 30% of cancer deaths,[5-10] 17 to 30% of cardiovascular deaths,[7,10-16] 30% of lung deaths,[7,10] 24% of pneumonia and influenza deaths,[17] 10% of infant deaths,[17,18] and 20 to 30% of low-birth-weight infants.[19,20] Approximately 3,000 lung cancer deaths annually among nonsmokers have been attributed to environmental tobacco smoke.[21] The total estimate from these causes formed the basis of 400,000 deaths in 1990 (Table 1).

MORTALITY FROM ALCOHOL

The prevalence of alcoholism in the U.S. was determined to be approximately 16% or 40 million people in the general population (Epidemiological Catchment Area Study–ECA data). While the use of alcohol contributes to an annual rate of approximately 100,000 deaths, the related health, social, and economic consequences from alcohol use results in additional costs of approximately 100 billion dollars a year. Alcohol use and alcoholism contributed to 60% to 90% of cirrhosis deaths,[22] 40% to 50% of motor vehicle fatalities,[12,23,24] 16% to 67% of home injuries, drownings, fire fatalities, and job injuries,[7,23,25] and 3% to 5% of cancer deaths.[6,7,9] The Carter Center project estimated that 5% of deaths and 15% of potential years of life were lost before age 65 because of alcohol use and alcoholism.[26] The CDC reported in 1987 that a total of 105,095 deaths were caused by alcohol, of which 30,000 deaths were from unintentional injuries, 19,600 from digestive diseases including liver cirrhosis, 17,700 from intentional injuries, and 16,000 from cancers (including those caused by tobacco).[27]

COSTS TO SOCIETY

The total health care costs in 1993 for the U.S. were approximately $900 billion,[28] or an average cost of more than $14,000 annually for a family of four. The magnitude of the contributions of the three leading causes of addictive illnesses (tobacco, alcohol, and other drugs) are clearly evident in the costs to society to treat the consequences of these addictive diseases. The expenditure on the treatment of the root causes, namely, prevention and treatment, of addictive illness was only a fraction of the total costs to individuals and society due to mortality and morbidity from addictive illnesses. The estimated expenditure for treatment of addictive illness was $20 billion and prevention was $5 billion in 1993.[1]

THE PREDICTORS OF MORTALITY IN ALCOHOLISM

Many studies have documented premature deaths or increased mortality among alcoholics and drug addicts.[3,29-37] The death rates and mortality ratios vary from two to six times the average for deaths in the U.S. population. Longitudinal studies show that alcoholics die 10-15 years earlier than members of the general population.[38] The highest rates for excess mortality are due to violent deaths, including suicide, homicide, accidents, and major diseases such as cardiovascular, cancer, hepatic, and pulmonary. Men have higher rates for early deaths than women because of greater rates of addictive illness, and complications and contributing diseases associated with mortality from alcoholism.

A recent study of predictors of mortality was conducted in a large, middle-aged (55 years of age and older), alcohol- and drug-addicted sample of Veterans' Administration patients.[39] They reported that older age, unmarried status, alcohol psychosis, organic brain disorder, medical illness (neoplasms, liver cirrhosis, and respiratory, endocrine, metabolic, and hematological disorders), and medical treatment (extended care facility residence, medical hospitalization, and medical treatment) contributed to increased mortality. Outpatient mental health treatment and posttreatment remission contributed to decreased mortality.[39]

THE ROLE OF ALCOHOL CONSUMPTION

Alcoholic cirrhosis is the ninth leading cause of death among all causes of death in the U.S. In general, the fluctuation in rates of cirrhosis has followed the per capita alcohol consumption over the past several decades. While alcoholic cirrhosis is a direct cause of death, indirect causes of death also have followed per capita alcohol consumption. Alcohol-related fatal traffic crashes, particularly among young people, remains a significant cause of death. In a study of 19 countries around the world having more than 200 motor vehicles per 1,000 population, the per capita alcohol consumption accounted for 70% of the variability in the death rates from vehicular accidents. Moreover, there was a direct association between alcohol consumption and vehicular deaths as both were reduced by the same amount during the 7-year period of the study.[40,41]

THE EFFECT OF ABSTINENCE ON MORTALITY AND TOBACCO USE IN ALCOHOLICS

Several studies showed that abstinence had a positive effect on the overall survival of alcoholics. Alcoholics who abstained from alcohol, particularly continuously, showed reduced mortality and increased years of longevity than those alcoholics who relapsed to alcohol consumption. The sources of the findings tend to be derived from treatment populations, where abstinence is expected to occur in higher rates than in the general population.[4,42,43]

A recent study of mortality examined alcoholics who were recruited from a treatment population of alcoholics for a prospective study of neurocognitive effects of alcoholism. A comparison on mortality was made between alcoholics who had achieved continuous abstinence and those alcoholics who had relapsed to alcohol. The sample of alcoholics was selected from a San Diego VA treatment program and/or members of local groups of Alcoholics Anonymous.[42] The original sample consisted of 234 alcoholic men who met DSM-III criteria for alcohol dependence, and the status of relapse and mortality was found in follow-up for 199 subjects (85%). Of these, 101 had relapsed and 98 had abstained. The same follow-up data were found for 92 of 98 matched control subjects (94%). There were 19 deaths among the relapsed alcoholics compared to 4 deaths in the abstinent alcoholics. The standardized mortality ratio for relapsed alcoholics was 4.96, and was significantly greater than 1.25 for the abstinent alcoholics which equaled that expected for the general population. The relapsed and abstinent alcoholics did not differ on other variables, such as demographic, medical, cognitive or prior drinking histories. The authors concluded that early mortality appeared significantly related to resumed drinking, and abstinent alcoholics recaptured survival rates comparable to those in the general U.S. population.[42]

The authors considered smoking but concluded that it lacked influence on the differences in mortality between the two alcoholic groups because: (1) The abstinent alcoholics smoked substantially more (8.1 packs/week vs. 2.2 packs/week) than the control group despite similar mortality rates. (2) The relapsed alcoholics smoked the same as abstinent alcoholics but had significantly higher mortality rates. (3) The smoking history was not significantly related to mortality in the Cox survival analysis. Death was ascertained from a variety of sources including collateral informants, state agencies, and the National Death Index.[42]

A study of mortality was conducted at 2-year and 8-year outcome following admission to a standard addiction treatment program for alcoholics and drug addicts.[43] Excessive mortality was found in the study population where there were 5.5 times as many deaths than expected in the general population matched for age, race, and gender. Moreover, alcoholics had higher mortality rates than drug addicts but that was attributed to the older age of the alcoholics. Excess deaths were found entirely among those whose alcoholism or drug use continued after treatment (or relapsed). At both 2 and 8 years later, the total number of deaths were significantly greater than expected from disease and other causes. The authors concluded that the most important finding from this study was the clear demonstration that recovery (absence of alcohol and drug use) from illness lengthened life from what was expected for active alcohol and drug use in addictive illness.

The study did not examine the effect of smoking as tobacco-related causes of death were not listed among the causes of death, namely, cardiovascular, peptic ulcer, liver disease, violence (accidents, suicides, homicides), and ingestions. Multiple sources were used in determining deaths including death certificates, autopsy, toxicology, hospital, police and other official records, and personal associates.[43]

A study of mortality during a 48-month follow-up in a group of 1,410 alcoholics who had received inpatient treatment showed similar benefits of abstinence from alcohol and drugs.[32] The patients who abstained from alcohol after 6 months had a mortality rate that was a third (4.4%) of that for the patients who had relapsed (12.4%) to alcohol/drugs. Patients who took drugs during the 18-month follow-up period had higher mortality rates; drugs listed were sleeping pills, 9.6%, psychoactive drugs, 9.7%, analgesics, 10.7%. The overall mortality rate for the four years was 7.6%, and twice as high among men as women (9.8% vs. 4.8%). The mortality rate increased with age, and the death rate in the sample was eight times that of men in the general population.[32] For both sexes, the standardized mortality ratio was highest at ages 20-29 and 30-39, and was similar overall for men and women. The variable abstinence/relapse contributed most to the probability of survival at the 48-month follow-up. Tobacco-related causes of death were not listed.[32]

THE ROLE OF TOBACCO USE IN ALCOHOLISM

The role of tobacco in mortality of alcoholics is yet to be fully determined as studies only recently have begun to establish links between death and smoking in alcoholics and abstinent alcoholics. As many as 90% of active alcoholics are smokers, and 30% of smokers can be diagnosed as alcoholics. Smoking is sufficiently strongly predictive of alcoholism that it should trigger a screen for an assessment of alcoholic drinking.[44-47]

However, the contribution of tobacco to mortality in alcoholics remains to be determined more fully. In a recent study, while the role of tobacco was strongly supported, alcoholism itself remained the greatest contributor to mortality. In a retrospective study of 845 treated alcoholics in Olmstead County in Minnesota, the cause of mortality was determined by death certificates from 1972 to 1983. No other confirmation of cause of death was included. The relative risk of dying from all causes was 2.6 (excess mortality greater than 1.0), alcohol-related was 4.1, tobacco-related was 2.0, alcohol–but not tobacco–related was 4.3, tobacco–but not alcohol–related was 1.8, related to both alcohol and tobacco was 1.4, and neither alcohol- nor tobacco-related was 4.2. Other significant causes of death included cancer, nutritional, cardiovascular disease, gastrointestinal disease, accidents, and suicides.[4]

While the importance of tobacco was substantiated, the relative risk for death from other causes remained high. Male gender and age (older) were associated with greater mortality but interestingly, lung cancer was not a significant contributor to death. Moreover, the smoking status at admission did predict mortality. A major weakness of the study was the lack of outcome data on multiple sources of documented causes of death as found in previous studies. The study did not include the patterns of use of alcohol, tobacco, or other drugs. The study did not provide information regarding effects of abstinence from tobacco on mortality or effects of abstinence from alcohol and other drugs on smoking behavior. Also, death certificates were obtained retrospectively, and no collateral information regarding causes of death was included. Death certificates alone may have underreported alcohol as an underlying cause of death (because of stigma and lack of acceptance of alcoholism as a disease).[4]

In a large primary prevention trial in 7,495 middle-aged men, smoking nonalcoholic men had a relative risk of dying almost double that of nonalcoholic nonsmokers. Among the nonsmoking alcoholics the risk of dying was three times and, in smoking alcoholics, over four times that of the nonalcoholic nonsmokers.[48]

In a prospective study of 9,889 males, a sample of 4,948 was examined for causes of death due to cancers and for separation of the effects of drinking and smoking on the cancer mortality of the alcoholic. The mortality of the alcoholic sample was compared to a sample of nonalcoholics which was matched according to smoking status. For specific causes, the rate of death from cancer of the lung and bronchus of the alcoholics was very similar to nonalcoholics, indicating heavy smoking as the cause. However, excess mortality from cancers of the head and neck remained high when smoking was controlled for, indicating an interaction between alcohol and smoking on mortality.[49]

A major reason why tobacco is not commonly cited as a cause of death among alcoholics more often is the age of onset of respiratory diseases caused by tobacco, e.g., bronchogenic cancer and chronic obstructive lung disease. The premature deaths due to alcoholism may preclude the onset of these respiratory causes of death in later life.

THE EFFECT OF COMORBIDITY ON MORTALITY

Standardized mortality ratios for psychiatric illness derived from comparisons with the general population and matched control groups have repeatedly shown excess mortality from both natural and unnatural causes among psychiatric patients.[50] Alcohol- and drug-related disorders including nicotine, alone or in combination with other psychiatric disorders have been repeatedly found to lead to increased mortality rates. Other psychiatric disorders that carry increased mortality rates include schizophrenia, organic brain disorder, mania, antisocial personality disorder. Interestingly, excess mortality is not always found with primary affective disorder (depression). The unnatural causes include suicide, homicide and accidents, whereas the natural causes include cerebrovascular, pulmonary, cerebrovascular, infectious diseases and others. However, death due to malignant neoplasms among psychiatric patients has not been found to be consistently higher than death due to these causes in the general population in the U.S.[50-52]

SUMMARY

The mortality from cigarette smoking and alcohol addiction is high. The combination of nicotine and alcohol use is common. The contributions to mortality from nicotine and alcohol are independent and additive depending on the associated cause of death. The recent documentation of increased mortality from tobacco smoking in otherwise abstinent alcoholics is important for clinicians to use to advise treated alcoholic patients with continued nicotine addiction. The documentation of reduced mortality in alcoholics following abstinence from tobacco smoking is yet to be determined.

REFERENCES

1. McGinnis JM, Foege WH: Actual causes of death in the United States. Journal of the American Medical Association 270(18):2207-2212, 1993.

2. National Center for Health Statistics. Health, U.S., 1992. Hyattsville, MD: U.S. Dept. of Health and Human Services Publication PHS 93-1232; 1993.

3. Lewis CE, Smith E, Kercher C, Spitznagel E: Predictors of mortality in alcoholic men: a 20-year follow-up study. Alcoholism: Clinical and Experimental Research 19(4):984-991, 1995.

4. Hurt RD, Offord KP, Croghan IT, Gomez-Dahl L, Kottke TE, Morse RM, Melton LJ: Mortality following inpatient addictions treatment: role of tobacco use in a community-based cohort. The Journal of the American Medical Association 275(14):1097-1103, 1996.

5. Rothenberg R, Nasca P, Mikl J, Burnett W, Reynolds B: Cancer. American Journal of Preventive Medicine 3(suppl):30-42, 1987.

6. Doll R, Peto R: The Causes of Cancer: Quantitative Estimates of Avoidable Risks of Cancer in the United States Today. New York, NY: Oxford University Press; 1981.

7. Milio N: Promoting Health Through Public Policy. Philadelphia, PA: F.A. Davis Co. Publishers; 1981.

8. Wynder EL, Gori G: Contribution of the environment to cancer incidence: an epidemiologic exercise. Journal of the National Cancer Institute 58:825-832, 1977.

9. Higginson J, Muir CS: Environmental carcinogenesis: misconceptions and limitations to cancer control. Journal of the National Cancer Institute 63: 1291-1298, 1979.

10. Gori GB, Richter BJ: Macroeconomics of disease prevention in the United States: prevention of major causes of mortality would alter life table assumptions and economic projections. Science 200:1124-1130, 1978.

11. White CC, Tolsma DD, Haynes SG, McGee D: Cardiovascular disease. American Journal of Preventive Medicine 3(suppl):43-54, 1987.

12. U.S. Preventive Services Task Force. Guide to Clinical Preventive Services: An Assessment of the Effectiveness of 169 Interventions. Baltimore, MD: Williams & Wilkins; 1989.

13. Goldman L, Cook EF: The decline in ischemic heart disease mortality rates: an analysis of the comparative effects of medical interventions and changes in lifestyle. Annals of Internal Medicine 101:825-836, 1984.

14. Paffenbarger RS, Hyde RT, Hsieh C, Wing AL: Physical activity, other life-style patterns, cardiovascular disease and longevity. Acta Medica Scandinavica 711(suppl):85-91, 1986.

15. Smith ESO: The economic impact of preventable ischemic heart disease. Canadian Medical Association Journal 117:507-512, 1977.

16. Manson JE, Tosteson H, Satterfield S, et al.: The primary prevention of myocardial infarction. The New England Journal of Medicine 326:1406-1416, 1992.

17. Centers for Disease Control and Prevention: Cigarette-attributable mortality and years of potential life lost–United States, 1990. MMWR Morbidity and Mortality Weekly Report 42:645-649, 1993.

18. Kleinman JC, Pierre MB, Madans JH, Land GH, Schramm WF: The effects of maternal smoking on fetal and infant mortality. American Journal of Epidemiology 127:274-282, 1988.

19. Kleinman JC, Madans JH: The effects of maternal smoking, physical stature, and educational attainment on the incidence of low birth weight. American Journal of Epidemiology 121:843-854, 1985.

20. The National Commission to Prevent Infant Mortality. Troubling Trends Persist: Shortchanging America's Next Generation. Washington, DC: U.S. Environmental Protection Agency; The National Commission to Prevent Infant Mortality; March 1992.

21. U.S. Environmental Protection Agency. Respiratory Health Effects of Passive Smoking, Lung Cancer and Other Disorders. Washington, DC: 1992. U.S. Environmental Protection Agency Publication 600/6-90/006F.

22. Johannes RS, Kahane SN, Mendeloff AI, Kurata J, Roth HP: Digestive diseases. American Journal of Preventive Medicine 3(suppl):83-88, 1987.

23. West LJ, Maxwell DS, Noble EP, Solomon DH: Alcoholism. Annals of Internal Medicine 100:405-416, 1984.

24. McCoy GF, Johnstone RA, Nelson IW, Duthie RB: A review of fatal road accidents in Oxfordshire over a 2-year period. Injury 20:65-68, 1989.

25. Smith GS, Falk H: Unintentional injuries. American Journal of Preventive Medicine 3(suppl):143-163, 1987.

26. Amler RW, Eddins DL: Cross-sectional analysis: precursors of premature death in the United States. American Journal of Preventive Medicine 3(supp.): 181-187, 1987.

27. Centers for Disease Control: Alcohol-related mortality and years of potential life lost–United States, 1987. MMWR Morbidity and Mortality Weekly Report 39:173-178, 1990.

28. Burner ST, Waldo DR, McKusick DR: National health expenditures projections through 2030. Health Care Financial Review 14:1-15, 1992.

29. U.S. Department of Health and Human Services: Eighth Special Report to the U.S. Congress on Alcohol and Health. National Institutes of Health, National Institute on Alcohol Abuse and Alcoholism. EEI, Alexandria, Virginia, contract no. ADM-281-91-0003, September 1993.

30. Stinson FS, DeBakey SF: Alcohol-related mortality in the United States, 1979-1988. British Journal of Addiction 87:777-783, 1992.

31. Finney JW, Moos RH: The long-term course of treated alcoholism: I. Mortality, relapse and remission rates and comparisons with community controls. Journal of Studies on Alcohol 52(1):44-54, 1991.

32. Feuerlein W, Küfner H, Flohrschütz T: Mortality in alcoholic patients given inpatient treatment. Addiction 89:841-849, 1994.

33. Marshall EJ, Edwards G, Taylor C: Mortality in men with drinking problems: a 20-year follow-up. Addiction 89:1293-1298, 1994.

34. Gillis LS: The mortality rate and causes of death of treated chronic alcoholics. South African Medical Journal 49:230-232, 1969.

35. Finney JW, Moos RH: The long-term course of treated alcoholism. II. Predictors and correlates of 10-year functioning and mortality. Journal of Studies on Alcohol 53:142-153, 1992.

36. Mackenzie A, Allen RP, Funderburk FR: Mortality and illness in male alcoholics: An 8-year follow-up. International Journal of the Addictions 21:865-882, 1986.

37. Ågren G, Romelsjö A: Mortality in alcohol-related diseases in Sweden during 1971-80 in relation to occupation, marital status, and citizenship in 1970. Scandinavian Journal of Social Medicine 20:134-142, 1992.

38. Schuckit MA: Treatment of alcoholism in office and outpatient settings. In Mendelson JH, Mello NK, eds. Medical Diagnosis and Treatment of Alcoholism. New York: McGraw Hill, Inc., 1992, pp. 363-392.

39. Moos RH, Brennan PL, Mertens JR: Mortality rates and predictors of mortality among late-middle-aged and older substance abuse patients. Alcoholism: Clinical and Experimental Research 18:187-195, 1994.

40. Smart RG, Mann RE: Alcohol and the epidemiology of liver cirrhosis. Alcohol Health and Research World 16:217-222, 1992.

41. Crabb DW, Lumeng L: Alcoholic liver diseases. In Kelley WN, DeVita VT, DuPont HL, Harris ED, Hazzard WR, Holmes EW, Hudson LD, Humes HD, Paty DW, Watanabe AM, Yamada T (eds): The Textbook of Internal Medicine. Philadelphia, PA. J.B. Lippincott Company, 1989, pp. 592-602.

42. Bullock KD, Reed RJ, Grant I: Reduced mortality risk: In alcoholics who achieve long-term abstinence. The Journal of the American Medical Association 267(5):668-672, 1992.

43. Barr HL, Antes D, Ottenberg DJ, Rosen A: Mortality of treated alcoholics and drug addicts: the benefits of abstinence. Journal of Studies on Alcohol 45(5):440-452, 1984.

44. Kozlowski LT, Skinner W, Kent C, Pope MA: Prospects for smoking treatment in individuals seeking treatment for alcohol and other drug problems. Addictive Behaviors 14:273-278, 1989.

45. Kozlowski LT, Wilkinson A, Skinner W, Kent C, Franklin T, Pope M: Comparing tobacco cigarette dependence with other drug dependencies. The Journal of the American Medical Association 261(6):898-901, 1989.

46. Burling TA, Ziff DC: Tobacco smoking: a comparison between alcohol and drug abuse inpatients. Addictive Behaviors 13:185-190, 1988.

47. Craig TJ, Van Natta PA: The association of smoking and drinking habits in a community sample. Journal of Studies on Alcohol 38(7):1434-1439, 1977.

48. Rosengren A, Wilhelmsen L, Wedel H: Separate and combined effects of smoking and alcohol abuse in middle-aged men. Acta Medica Scandinavica 223:111-118, 1988.

49. Schmidt W, Popham RE: The role of drinking and smoking in mortality from cancer and other causes in male alcoholics. Cancer 47:1031-1041, 1981.

50. Felker B, Yazel JJ, Short D: Mortality and medical comorbidity among psychiatric patients: a review. Psychiatric Services 47(12):1356-1363, 1996.

51. West LJ, Maxwell DS, Noble EP, Solomon DH: Alcoholism. UCLA Conference. Annals of Internal Medicine 100:405-416, 1984.

52. Edwards G, Duckitt A, Oppenheimer E, Sheehan M, Taylor C: What happens to alcoholics? The Lancet 30:269-271, July 30, 1983.

Tobacco, Alcohol, and Drug Use in a Primary Care Sample: 90-Day Prevalence and Associated Factors

Linda Baier Manwell, BS
Michael F. Fleming, MD
Kristen Johnson, MA
Kristen Lawton Barry, PhD

SUMMARY. Background: Primary care settings are an ideal system in which to identify and treat substance use disorders.

Objective: To ascertain the prevalence of tobacco, alcohol, and drug use in the office of 88 primary care clinicians by gender, age and ethnicity.

Method: 21,282 adults ages 18-65 completed a self-administered Health Screening Survey while participating in a trial for early alcohol treatment.

Linda Baier Manwell is Deputy Director, Center for Addiction Research and Education; Michael F. Fleming is Director, Center for Addiction Research and Education and Associate Professor, Department of Family Medicine; and Kristen Johnson is Programmer Analyst, Center for Addiction Research and Education, University of Wisconsin-Madison, Madison, WI.

Kristen Lawton Barry is Associate Research Scientist, Department of Psychiatry, University of Michigan, Ann Arbor, MI.

Address correspondence to: Linda Baier Manwell, BS, Center for Addiction Research and Education, 777 South Mills Street, Madison, WI 53715

This work was supported by the NIAAA-grant number R01 AA08512-02 and the Wisconsin Research Network (WReN).

[Haworth co-indexing entry note]: "Tobacco, Alcohol, and Drug Use in a Primary Care Sample: 90-Day Prevalence and Associated Factors." Manwell, Linda Baier et al. Co-published simultaneously in *Journal of Addictive Diseases* (The Haworth Medical Press, an imprint of The Haworth Press, Inc.) Vol. 17, No. 1, 1998, pp. 67-81; and: *Smoking and Illicit Drug Use* (ed: Mark S. Gold, and Barry Stimmel) The Haworth Medical Press, an imprint of The Haworth Press, Inc., 1998, pp. 67-81. Single or multiple copies of this article are available for a fee from The Haworth Document Delivery Service [1-800-342-9678, 9:00 a.m. - 5:00 p.m. (EST). E-mail address: getinfo@haworth.com].

Results: The period prevalence of tobacco use was 27%. For alcohol: abstainers 40%, low risk drinkers 38%, at-risk drinkers 9%, problem drinkers 8%, and dependent drinkers 5%. Twenty percent of the sample reported using illicit drugs five or more times in their lifetime and 5% reported current illicit drug use. There were marked differences in alcohol use disorders by age and ethnicity. The majority of persons who smoked reported the desire to cut down or stop using tobacco.

Significance: This is the first report on the combined prevalence of tobacco, alcohol and drug disorders in a large sample of persons attending community-based non-academic primary care clinics. This report confirms the high prevalence of these problems and suggests that patients will accurately complete a self-administered screening test such as the Health Screening Survey. The office procedures developed for this study provide Managed Care Organizations with a system of care that can be used to screen all persons for tobacco, alcohol and drug use disorders. *[Article copies available for a fee from The Haworth Document Delivery Service: 1-800-342-9678. E-mail address: getinfo@haworth.com]*

INTRODUCTION

Tobacco, alcohol, and drug use disorders are among the most common problems seen in primary care. Twenty-five percent of U.S. adults use tobacco products–chewing tobacco, snuff, cigars, cigarettes, and pipe tobacco–on a regular basis. In the U.S. alone, 435,000 deaths are attributable to tobacco use annually.[1] Cigarette smoking is the leading cause of preventable morbidity and mortality in the United States.[2] Diseases attributable to smoking include cancer (lip, oral cavity, larynx, esophagus, pharynx, lung, bladder, pancreas, kidney), chronic obstructive lung disease, and cardiovascular disease. Smoking has been implicated in adverse outcomes of pregnancy including low birth weight and intrauterine growth retardation. Exposure to second-hand smoke is associated with asthma, an increased number of upper respiratory infections, lung cancer, decreased pulmonary function, and cardiovascular disease in non-smokers.[3]

Alcohol use is also associated with adverse health effects including liver cirrhosis, cancer, cardiovascular disease, depression, and trauma. Many of these effects are causally related to the quantity and pattern of alcohol use. For example, the relative risk of liver cirrhosis, based on a pooled estimate of the published research, is 2.2 for males who drink greater than 20 grams of alcohol per day[4] (one standard U.S. drink contains 12-14 grams of alcohol). Women seem to be more susceptible to liver cirrhosis than men.[5,6] Cancers associated with alcohol use include oropharyngeal, esophageal, hepatic, and breast.[7,8,9,10] A number of studies have found a dose-response effect between stroke mortality and alcohol consumption.[11,12]

Illicit drug use is associated with overdose, acquired immune deficiency syndrome (AIDS), other infections (cellulitis, hepatitis, endocarditis), and trauma such as falls, burns, suicides, homicides, and motor vehicle accidents. Babies exposed to drugs in utero can suffer fetal death or other severe effects including growth retardation, organ damage, cognitive defects, and behavioral problems.[13] In addition, more than one-half of reported cases of child abuse and neglect involve drug abuse by the parents.[14]

While the National Household Survey[15] provides general population estimates on the prevalence of these problems, there is limited data from primary care practices. The purpose of this paper is to present the results of a prevalence study conducted in the offices of 88 primary care physicians in Wisconsin. Predictive factors for substance abuse are identified utilizing information gathered through the use of a health questionnaire querying various physical and mental health issues.

METHODS

The study was conducted in the offices of 88 primary care physicians at 22 sites who had agreed to participate in an early intervention alcohol treatment project (Project TrEAT: Trial for Early Alcohol Treatment). A Health Screening Survey (HSS) was offered to all patients ages 18 through 65 with regularly scheduled appointments between April 1, 1992 and April 1, 1994. The clinics were located in rural and urban areas in south central and southeastern Wisconsin and varied from solo practices to large HMO groups. The methodology and results of this trial are reported elsewhere.[16]

The HSS, validated in two treatment samples and one primary care sample,[17] was based on a scale originally developed by Wallace and Haines.[18] It was designed as a general lifestyle questionnaire in order to increase patient acceptance of the research procedures and to minimize the intervention effect of the alcohol questions. The office staff at each of the clinics received standardized training regarding research procedures and questionnaire dissemination. Research assistants worked in each of the clinics to ensure appropriate completion of the study procedures.

The HSS included four sets of parallel questions regarding exercise, cigarette use, alcohol use, and weight control. The tobacco section inquired about use during the past three months and the average number of cigarettes smoked each day. Four questions modified from the alcohol CAGE questions[19] were included: (1) "In the last 3 months, have you felt you should cut down or stop smoking?"; (2) "In the last 3 months, has anyone annoyed you or got on your nerves by telling you to cut down or stop smoking?"; (3) In the last 3 months, have you felt guilty or bad about how much you smoke?"; and (4) "In the last 3 months, have you been waking up in the morning wanting to smoke a cigarette?". The final smoking-related question inquired about whether the patient believed that he/she EVER had a smoking problem. This question was based on the clinical observation that patients are more willing to admit to a past than a present problem.

Four sections on alcohol use were included on the HSS. The first section asked patients if they had consumed any alcoholic beverages during the past three months. Those who responded in the affirmative were asked more detailed consumption questions regarding the quantity and frequency of beer, wine, or liquor consumed per week during the three-month period. For each of three categories of beverages, examples were cited and respondents were asked "on average" the number of days per week the beverage was consumed and the number of glasses, bottles, or cans consumed on one day by marking the appropriate category. Alcohol consumption was tabulated as an average number of drinks/week for the three types of alcohol consumed.

The second alcohol use section on the HSS queried the number of episodes of binge drinking, determined by a question about the number of times the patient had six or more drinks on one occasion in the past three months. Categorical responses included: none, one-two, three-five, and more than five. The third section, the four-item CAGE questionnaire,[19] was also included. Subjects were asked: "In the last three months have you felt you should cut down on your drinking?" "Has anyone annoyed you by telling you to cut down or stop your drinking?" "Have you felt guilty or bad about your drinking?" "Have you been waking up in the morning wanting to have an alcoholic drink?"

The fourth section asked for patients' perceptions as to whether they had a past or present alcohol problem. This is based on the clinical observation that patients are more willing to admit to a past than a present problem, and that admission of a past problem is significantly related to having a present alcohol problem.

A randomly-selected 10% subsample received an extended Health Screening Survey (HSS-B) to collect data on other factors shown in the literature to be associated with alcohol disorders. These included questions regarding use of other mood-altering drugs, family history of alcohol or drug problems, and questions from the Diagnostic Interview Schedule (DIS)[20] developed for identifying probable depression, conduct disorder, and antisocial personality disorder. The drug use section focused on the frequency of drug use in the previous 6 months including use of cannabinoids, amphetamines, sedatives, cocaine or crack, heroin, other opiates, psychedelics, and inhalants.

The Health Screening Surveys were distributed to patients upon arrival by reception staff and collected in a locked box prior to departure. The patients' medical records were coded so that patients only received the survey once. Research assistants visited the clinics at least twice a week to collect the surveys and interview clinic personnel to ascertain problems. The rate of patient refusal varied by clinic with a range of 2%-30% and a weighted mean of 13% for a 87% response rate. The most common reasons given for refusal were lack of time or feeling too ill to complete the survey. Data from completed surveys were read by an optical scanner into a computerized data base.

Data were summarized and statistically analyzed using SPSS[x]. Frequency distributions and summary statistics were calculated for variables of interest. Analyses were carried out separately for males and females as well as selected age groups and ethnic groups. Gender differences for all categorical data were then analyzed using Mantel Hanzel chi square, adjusting for age.

RESULTS

The Health Screening Survey was completed by 21,282 adults. Two-thirds of the population were female with a mean age of 41. While the majority of the subjects were Caucasian, 679 African Americans and 368 persons of Hispanic descent completed the survey. Nearly a quarter of the sample graduated from college. Three quarters were married or living with a partner. Over 80% of the sample were employed outside the home with no significant difference by gender. The majority lived in a household with two or more persons.

Smoking Prevalence

The overall frequency of cigarette use was similar to findings from the *National Household Survey*.[15] Tables 1 and 2 present smoking prevalence data. Twenty-seven percent of the sample reported cigarette use in the previous three months with no gender differences. About 8% of those who

TABLE 1. Frequency of Cigarette Use and Smoking CAGE 90-Day Prevalence (By Age)

	Ages 18-30	Ages 31-50	Ages 51-65	p value	Total
Total sample size by age	(n = 4,882)	(n = 10,967)	(n = 5,353)		(n = 21,202)
Cigarette use in last 90 days (any use)	32.6%	27.5%	19.2%	.0001	26.6%
Total sample smoking in past 90 days (by age)	(n = 1,558)	(n = 2,968)	(n = 989)		(n = 5,536)
Of those who smoked in past 90 days, number of cigarettes/day					
<1	12.3%	6.5%	4.5%		7.9%
1-9	30.5%	24.3%	26.2%		26.4%
10-19	32.9%	30.2%	31.8%		31.2%
>20	24.3%	39.0%	37.6%	.0001	34.5%
Of those who smoked in past 90 days, perceived smoking as a problem	69.8%	83.6%	84.3%	.0001	79.8%
Of those who smoked in past 90 days, felt should cut down	84.4%	90.9%	89.5%	.0001	88.8%
Of those who smoked in past 90 days, woke up wanting to smoke	66.6%	73.3%	71.1%	.0001	71.0%

TABLE 2. Frequency of Cigarette Use and Smoking CAGE 90-Day Prevalence (By Ethnicity)

	Caucasian	Asian-Amer	Hispanic	Native Amer	African-Amer	Other	p value
Total sample	(n = 18,151)	(n = 202)	(n = 363)	(n = 161)	(n = 673)	(n = 552)	
Cigarette use last 90 days							
	25.7%	22.3%	24.0%	42.2%	42.2%	28.1%	.0001
Total sample who smoked last 90 days							
	(n = 4,602)	(n = 43)	(n = 86)	(n = 66)	(n = 276)	(n = 153)	
Of those who smoked in past 90 days, number of cigarettes/day							
<1	7.4%	13.6%	23.5%	11.3%	6.1%	10.0%	
1-9	24.2%	31.8%	42.4%	37.1%	52.7%	31.3%	
10-19	32.0%	31.8%	21.2%	12.9%	26.5%	31.3%	
>19	36.3%	22.7%	12.9%	38.7%	14.8%	27.3%	.0001
Of those who smoked in past 90 days, perceived smoking as a problem							
	81.1%	73.3%	57.8%	72.3%	77.2%	69.6%	.0001
Of those who smoked in past 90 days, felt should cut down							
	89.2%	86.0%	77.6%	89.6%	89.7%	85.7%	.0196
Of those who smoked in past 90 days, woke up wanting to smoke							
	71.0%	72.7%	50.0%	56.7%	80.9%	71.0%	.0001

smoked cigarettes in the last three months smoked less than one cigarette per day. Twenty-six percent reported smoking one to nine cigarettes per day. Mean cigarette use was 13 cigarettes per day. The largest smoking group were those who smoked one or more packs of cigarettes per day; 58% of the men and 48% of the women. The highest rates of smoking by age were in young persons (33% smoked in the previous 90 days), higher than the 29% reported in the *National Household Survey*. The lowest rates were in persons over the age of 50.

Table 2 presents smoking frequency by ethnicity. Noticeable differences were found in the five racial groups who participated in the survey. Native Americans and African-Americans had the highest percentage of smokers (42%) and Asian Americans had the lowest (22%). Native American males had the highest smoking rate, with fully 50% reporting cigarette use within the last 90 days. The percentage of smokers was evenly distributed between males and females in each race except for Native Americans (males 50%, females 39%).

Alcohol Prevalence

Prevalence data on alcohol use are presented in Tables 3 and 4. Forty percent of the sample had no alcohol to drink in the three months prior to the survey. About one-third were low-risk drinkers. The rest fell into the at-risk, problem, and dependent drinker categories, hereafter referred to as problematic drinking. The frequency of problematic drinking varied depending on the cut-off value chosen to define it. Using drinking limits recommended by the National Institute on Alcohol Abuse and Alcoholism (>14 drinks week for men, >7 drinks per week for women), the frequency of problematic drinking was 20% for men and 19% for women.

Minimal differences were found when looking at average weekly consumption by age. The highest rates of problematic drinking were in patients ages 18-30 (28%) and the lowest in subjects greater than age 50 (19%). Across all ages, men were more likely to be problematic drinkers than women. Of patients ages 18-30, men were nearly twice as likely to be at-risk drinkers and more than twice as likely to be dependent drinkers.

Further analysis of average drinking levels demonstrates that men drink significantly more than women. Men were three times more likely to drink three or more drinks per day than women, and were twice as likely to have engaged in binge drinking in the last three months (defined as 6 or more drinks on one occasion). Sixteen percent of men reported three or more episodes of binge drinking in the last 90 days, compared to only 4.5% of women.

Table 4 presents differences in the frequency of at-risk drinking by

TABLE 3. Frequency of Drinking Categories 90-Day Prevalence Estimate (By Gender and Age)

	Male			Female			Total by age			p value	Total*
Ages	18-30	31-50	51-65	18-30	31-50	51-65	18-30	31-50	51-65		
Sample size	(1472)	(4144)	(1322)	(3389)	(6809)	(3031)	(4892)	(11,012)	(5378)		(21,282)
Abstainers	25.7%	30.5%	39.0%	32.7%	43.5%	58.1%	30.7%	38.8%	49.9%	.0001	39.6%
Low risk users	46.8	45.2	37.8	38.9	35.1	25.5	41.1	38.8	30.7	.0001	37.7
At-risk users	4.6	4.4	4.5	17.4	12.0	10.6	13.5	9.1	7.9	.0001	9.4
Problem users	12.4	11.6	11.3	6.7	6.1	4.2	8.5	8.1	7.3	.0001	8.0
Dependent users	10.4	8.3	7.4	4.3	3.3	1.7	6.2	5.2	4.2	.0001	5.2

Abstainers: Less than one drink per month

Low risk users: Females 1-7 drinks/wk: males 1-14 drinks/wk

At-risk users: Females 8-21 drinks/wk; males 15-21 drinks/wk

Problem users: 22-35 drinks/wk and/or 2 positive CAGE

Dependent users: 3 or more positive CAGE and/or 5 or more drinks/day

* Totals may differ due to some patients' non-response to gender question.

TABLE 4. Frequency of Drinking Categories 90-Day Prevalence Estimate (By Ethnicity)

	Caucasian	Asian-Amer	Hispanic	Native Amer	African-Amer	Other	p value
sample size	(n = 18,151)	(n = 202)	(n = 363)	(n = 161)	(n = 673)	(n = 552)	
Abstainers	37.5%	53.7%	54.7%	48.4%	49.5%	53.0%	.0001
Low risk user	39.5	24.2	25.6	24.2	20.7	25.9	.0001
At-risk user	10.1	9.5	6.3	11.1	6.2	8.7	.0007
Problem user	8.1	7.9	7.4	8.5	9.9	5.7	.2381
Dependent	4.8	4.7	6.0	7.8	13.6	6.7	.0001

Abstainers: Less than one drink per month

Low risk users: Females 1-7 drinks/wk; males 1-14 drinks/wk

At-risk users: Females 8-21 drinks/wk; males 15-21 drinks/wk

Problem users: 22-35 drinks/wk and/or 2 positive CAGE

Dependent users: 3 or more positive CAGE and/or 5 or more drinks/day race/ethnicity using the drinking limits recommended by the National Institute on Alcohol Abuse and Alcoholism[21]. Some differences by race/ethnicity were noted, with Native American men having the highest rate of problematic use and Hispanic women the lowest. African-American and Native American groups had the highest overall rates of use.

Other Drug Prevalence

A 10% subsample (n = 1,928) of patients completed an extended Health Screening Survey (HSS-B) that included a section focusing on lifetime and current use (in the last six months) of drugs. Inquiries were made regarding the use of tranquilizers, sleeping pills, marijuana, stimulants, cocaine, narcotics, PCP, psychedelics, and inhalants. To assess lifetime use, patients were asked if they used any of these drugs more than five times in their lifetime to get high. Nineteen percent of the subsample reported using drugs in their lifetime; of these, 25.3% reported using drugs in the last six months.

Marijuana accounted for most of the illegal drug use. Of those who used drugs, 87.8% had used marijuana in their lifetime and 22.5% had used it in the last six months. Men had a higher frequency of lifetime use than women although the difference was not significant (p = .1258). Marijuana use was more prevalent among those 18-30 years of age (p = .0001 for lifetime use). Among the subsample who reported drug use, the second most frequently used drug was cocaine with a lifetime prevalence of 30.8% and a 6-month prevalence of 6.9%.

Of those who used drugs, 12% reported that they felt they have had a problem with drug use at some point in their lifetime. Men were more likely to report this than women (15% vs. 10%; p = .1604). Patients ages 18-30 also reported this more frequently (17% for 18-30, 10% for 31-50, 0% for 51- 65; p = .0312). Among ethnic groups, Hispanics reported a problem with drug use at some point in their lifetime most often (21%), followed in frequency by African-Americans (18%), and Caucasians (11%); however, these differences are were not significant (p = .6834).

Treatment Issues

As shown in Table 1, 80% of smokers in this survey felt that they had a problem with cigarettes, with no difference by gender. Eighty-nine percent felt that they should reduce their smoking, with no difference by gender or age. Native American males, who had the highest rate of smoking, also had the highest response rate when asked if they perceived smoking as a problem. These smokers realize smoking is a problem and that a reduction in use is warranted. Clinicians should be poised to facilitate smoking cessation for these patients. A question regarding tobacco use should be included as part of every clinic's vital signs. Offers of support for smoking cessation should be a routine part of every smoker's clinic visit and clinic personnel should be trained in tobacco cessation strategies. Office-based intervention in medical practices has been shown to be successful[22] and all staff members should be involved in the design of an intervention support system.

As noted in Table 3, 9% of the study sample fell into the at-risk drinking category and 8% were classified as problem drinkers. An Institute of Medicine report[23] suggests that the identification and treatment of at-risk users is at least as important as the identification and treatment of persons who are alcohol dependent. Clinicians need to shift away from the exclusive detection of alcoholism and move toward the recognition and treatment of at-risk and problem drinkers. The use of quantity/frequency questions, combined with the CAGE, are an effective means of screening patients for alcohol use. Once identified, at-risk and problem drinkers have been shown to respond positively to brief physician advice.[16] Brief advice treatment can also be used with dependent drinkers to overcome their unwillingness to seek treatment by helping them to move from pre-contemplation to action.

Almost one-fifth of the study subsample had used drugs more than five times in their lifetime to get high. Five percent were currently using drugs. Marijuana was the most-often used drug, especially by subjects 18-30 and males. Even though physician-delivered brief advice treatment is not commonly used in the primary care setting for illicit drug use, data from smoking and problem drinking trials indicate success with persons who have minimal as well as severe physiological dependence. The clinical experience of physicians working in primary care suggests that brief advice can be an effective method in changing drug use.[24] It can be used to assist patients to become abstinent as well as to convince patients who are reluctant to participate in a specialized treatment program. A trial by Roffman et al.[25] indicated that patients who received two sessions with a therapist regarding their marijuana use did as well as a group who received weekly care over a ten-week period. Future studies on brief intervention for illicit drug abuse will clarify the effectiveness of this treatment method.

DISCUSSION

This large-scale epidemiological survey of patients attending U.S. community-based primary care clinics provides a stable estimate of tobacco, alcohol, and drug use in over 21,000 adults ages 18-65. The findings of the survey have important implications for the U.S. health care system. As managed care systems continue to implement prevention programs to reduce the consequences and costs associated with substance abuse, they need prevalence estimates to allocate resources and services. Also, the identification of predictive factors may help primary care physicians to target specific populations within their practices and communities for prevention activities.

This study has a number of strengths. They include a large sample size, recruitment of subjects from a large number of community-based primary care practices, a high response rate, and the application of standardized questions and scales. The use of community-based physicians increases the external validity of the findings and allows comparison with community physician practices in other states. Study limitations include the use of a screening survey to estimate the quantity and pattern of substance use. Also, the generalizability of the findings of this study to primary care practices in other parts of the U.S. is not known.

In summary, the data presented in this paper suggest that in Wisconsin, 27% of adults seeking general medical care smoke cigarettes, 20% are at risk for alcohol related problems, and 5% are currently using drugs. This has a significant impact on health care resources. Physicians are currently expected to conduct and implement an increasing number of prevention activities including screening for hypertension, hypercholesterolemia, cancer, alcohol use, domestic violence, hyperglycemia, seat belt use, depression, etc. A simple screening tool such as the Health Screening Survey and the utilization of risk-factor assessment can help these physicians in their prevention efforts. The implementation of systematic screening and prevention activities for tobacco use can positively impact on patients' health status and their utilization of health care resources.

REFERENCES

1. Centers for Disease Control. Cigarette smoking–attributable mortality and years of potential life lost: United States, 1990. MMWR Morb Mortal Wkly Rep 1993;42:645-9.

2. Elixhauser A. The costs of smoking and the cost effectiveness of smoking cessation programs. J Public Health Policy. 1990;11:218-37.

3. U.S. Department of Health and Human Services. The health consequences of involuntary smoking: a report of the Surgeon General. Washington, DC: DHHS, Public Health Service, Office of the Assistant Secretary for Health, Office of Smoking and Health, 1986. DHHS publication no. PHS 87-8398.

4. Anderson P, Cremona A, Paton A, Turner C, Wallace P. The risk of alcohol. Addiction. 1993;88:1493-1508.

5. Tuyns AJ, Pequinot G. Greater risk of ascetic cirrhosis in females in relation to alcohol consumption. Int J Epidemiol. 1984;13:53-7.

6. Norton R, Batey R, Dyer T, MacMahon S. Alcohol consumption and the risk of alcohol-related cirrhosis in women. BMJ. 1987;295:80-2.

7. Tuyns AJ, Esteve J, Raymond L, et al. Cancer of the larynx/hypopharynx, tobacco, and alcohol. Int J Cancer. 1988;41:483-91.

8. Austin H, Delzell E, Grufferman S et al. A case-control study of hepatocellular carcinoma and the hepatitis B virus, cigarette smoking, and alcohol consumption. Cancer Res. 1986;46: 962-6.

9. Schatzkin A, Jones D, Hoover RN, et al. Alcohol consumption and breast cancer in the epidemiologic follow-up study of the first National Health and Nutrition Examination Survey. N Engl J Med. 1987;316:1169-73.

10. Willett WC, Stampfer MJ, Colditz GA, et al. Moderate alcohol consumption and the risk of breast cancer. N Engl J Med. 1987;316:1174-80.

11. Donahue RP, Abbott RD, Reed DM, Yano K. Alcohol and hemorrhagic stroke. The Honolulu Health Program. JAMA. 1986;255:2311-14.

12. Semenciw RM, Morrison HI, Mao Y, et al. Major risk factors for cardiovascular disease mortality in adults: Results from the Nutrition Canada Survey cohort. Int J Epidemiol. 1988;17:317-24.

13. Hoffman RS, Goldfrank LR. The impact of drug abuse and addiction on society. Emerg Med Clin North Am. 1990;8(3):467-80.

14. Select Committee on Narcotics Abuse and Control. On the edge of the American dream: a social and economic profile in 1992. A Report by the Chairman. Washington, DC: U.S. Government Printing Office, 1992.

15. U.S. Department of Health and Human Services. National household survey on drug abuse: population estimates 1993. Washington, DC: DHHS, Public Health Service, Substance Abuse and Mental Health Services Administration, 1994. DHHS publication no. (SMA) 94-3017.

16. Fleming MF, Barry KL, Baier Manwell L et al. Brief physician advice for problem alcohol drinkers: a randomized controlled tiral in community-based primary care practices. JAMA. 1997; 277:1039-1045.

17. Fleming M, Barry K. A three-sample test of an alcohol screening questionnaire. Alcohol Alcohol. 1991;26(1):81-91.

18. Wallace PG, Haines AP. The use of a questionnaire in general practice to increase the recognition of patients with excessive alcohol consumption. BMJ. 1985;290(6486):1949-53.

19. Ewing JA. Detecting alcoholism: the CAGE questionnaire. JAMA. 1984;252:1905-1907.

20. Robins LN, Helzer JE, Croughan JL, Ratcliff KS. National Institute of Mental Health Diagnostic Interview Schedule: Its history, characteristics, and validity. Arch Gen Psychiatry. 1981;38:381-9.

21. National Institute on Alcohol Abuse and Alcoholism. The physicians' guide to helping patients with alcohol problems. U.S. Department of Health and Human Services, Public Health Service, National Institutes of Health, NIAAA, 1995. NIH publication no. 95-3769.

22. Cummings SR, Coates TJ, Stein MS, Swan ND. Smoking cessation in primary care practices: summary of results from the Quit for Life Project. In: Tobacco and the clinician: interventions for medical and dental practice. Smoking and tobacco control. Monograph 5. Department of Health and Human Services, Public Health Service, National Institutes of Health, National Cancer Institute. Washington, DC: U.S. Government Printing Office. NIH Publication no. 94-3693. January, 1994.

23. Institute of Medicine, Division of Mental health and Behavioral Medicine. Broadening the base of treatment for alcohol problems. Washington, DC: National Academy Press, 1990.

24. Trachenberg R, Fleming MF. Diagnosis and Treatment of drug abuse in family practice. American Family Physician Monograph, Summer 1994.

25. Roffman RA, Stephens RS, Simpson EE, Whitaker DL. Treatment of marijuana dependence: preliminary results. J Psychoactive Drugs. 1988;20:129-37.

Incorporating Nicotine Dependence into Addiction Treatment

Terry A. Rustin, MD

SUMMARY. An addiction treatment program devoted two years to preparing to become a smokefree treatment unit that addressed nicotine dependence as another drug dependency. Data collected from September 1990 to July 1995 on 263 admissions before becoming smokefree and 2182 admissions after making the transition revealed that going smokefree did not affect the incidence of premature discharges or aggressive behavior, and did not change the overall rate of program completion by either smokers or nonsmokers. During the first three months after going smokefree, the program completion rate dropped for both smokers and nonsmokers; by the fourth month, it had returned to previous levels. Seventeen months after going smokefree, the program completion rate was higher than it had ever been. This suggests that the drop in the program completion rate was due to the disruption caused by a significant programmatic change and not due to the unit's smokefree status, and that the increasing experience of staff in treating nicotine dependence resulted in improved patient outcomes. *[Article copies available for a fee from The Haworth Document Delivery Service: 1-800-342-9678. E-mail address: getinfo@haworth.com]*

Terry A. Rustin is affiliated with the Department of Psychiatry and Behavioral Sciences, University of Texas Houston Medical School, Houston, TX.

Address correspondence to: Terry A. Rustin, MD, Director, Dual Disorders Programs, Mental Health and Mental Retardation Authority of Harris County, 2850 Fannin, Houston, TX 77002.

The author is grateful to Richard Chen, PhD, who calculated the statistics reported in this paper, and to the staff members of Unit 3B who made it possible. The staff members who led the nicotine dependence groups deserve special recognition: Rita Seelen, LCDC; Anndora Garner, RN; and Trevaine Rogers, RN.

[Haworth co-indexing entry note]: "Incorporating Nicotine Dependence into Addiction Treatment." Rustin, Terry A. Co-published simultaneously in *Journal of Addictive Diseases* (The Haworth Medical Press, an imprint of The Haworth Press, Inc.) Vol. 17, No. 1, 1998, pp. 83-108; and: *Smoking and Illicit Drug Use* (ed: Mark S. Gold, and Barry Stimmel) The Haworth Medical Press, an imprint of The Haworth Press, Inc., 1998, pp. 83-108. Single or multiple copies of this article are available for a fee from The Haworth Document Delivery Service [1-800-342-9678, 9:00 a.m. - 5:00 p.m. (EST). E-mail address: getinfo@haworth.com].

The reasonable man adapts himself to the world; the unreasonable one persists in trying to adapt the world to himself. Therefore, all progress depends on the unreasonable man.

George Bernard Shaw

INTRODUCTION

Substantial evidence supports the concept that nicotine produces tolerance (neuroadaptation), withdrawal signs and symptoms, characteristic drug-seeking behavior, and psychoactive effects,[1-4] and thus meets the criteria for being an addicting chemical. Further research suggests that nicotine dependence shares characteristics with other chemical dependencies.[5,6] Epidemiological research has established the comorbidity of nicotine dependence and other drug dependencies, and of nicotine dependence and psychiatric and emotional disorders.[7-15] Despite this evidence that nicotine is an addicting drug, addiction treatment centers and psychiatric units have been reluctant to incorporate nicotine dependence treatment modalities into their programs, often out of concern that patients would refuse admission, leave prematurely, or have a poorer outcome because nicotine dependence was addressed during treatment.[16-27]

Alina Lodge in New Jersey is generally recognized as the first addiction treatment program in the United States to insist that its patients stop using tobacco along with other drugs and alcohol.[28] Alina Lodge is a free-standing program in a rural area; its program reflects the charismatic personality of its director, Geraldine Delaney. This treatment center uses a firm, unambiguous 12-Step approach to treat patients who have been unable to maintain abstinence following multiple previous treatments elsewhere; Alina Lodge is considered the "treatment center of last resort" for alcoholics with a history of multiple relapses. Prospective clients of Alina Lodge who see it as their last resort have no choice but to accept its smokefree policies. Although Ms. Delaney's report[28] provided no outcome data, it encouraged others to proceed further.

The Veterans Administration Hospital in Minneapolis, Minnesota, became smokefree in June 1988;[29] however, their patients were afforded opportunities to smoke when not on the treatment unit. Today, all Veterans' Administration Hospitals provide smokefree treatment environments, but the degree to which they incorporate nicotine dependence into their addiction treatment programs varies widely.[30,31] Most VA treatment units permit patients relatively free access to outdoor areas where they can smoke during free time, and the programs do not attempt to control patient smoking behavior when patients are away from the hospital.

The addiction treatment program at CPC Parkwood Hospital in Atlanta became smokefree in October 1989. Under the leadership of Paul Earley and Michael Fishman, CPC Parkwood gradually incorporated more programming on nicotine dependence over a two year period; the new program gained acceptance from referral agencies and the community. Earley and Fishman left that facility in December 1991, and the medical leadership that replaced them did not share their commitment to nicotine dependence treatment. Under administrative pressure, the unit's policy reverted to its previous status; smoking was again permitted on the unit and attendance in nicotine dependence activities became optional (Paul Earley, personal communication).

Gateway Rehabilitation Center in Aliquippa, Pennsylvania became smokefree in 1989 under the leadership of its medical directors, Abraham Twerski and Neil Capretto.[32] Gateway is a large, free-standing treatment program which aggressively seeks referrals from Employee Assistance Programs and other referral sources. After a short period of planning, the facility and campus became smokefree, but without adequately addressing nicotine dependence in staff members and without developing a clear vision of the program as smokefree. Six months after going smokefree, with staff members, patients and referral sources actively sabotaging the nicotine dependence program, Gateway made its nicotine dependence program optional (Neil Capretto, personal communication.) The treatment program at the Medical College of Virginia in Richmond, Virginia, run by Sidney Schnoll and Lori Karan, had a fate similar to that of Gateway,[33] as did the efforts to go smokefree at Sierra Tucson in Tucson, Arizona (George Nash, personal communication).

The hospitals and clinics of the Mayo Clinic in Rochester, Minnesota have long been in the forefront of developing medical models of nicotine dependence treatment.[34] Following a process lasting several years, their psychiatric and addiction treatment services have now become smokefree and their staff members actively address nicotine dependence within the context of addiction treatment (Richard Finlayson, personal communication; Karen Schultz, personal communication).

Mindful of the potential problems reported by others, in July 1989 we set out to transform one of the two addiction treatment units of the Harris County Psychiatric Center in Houston, Texas into a smokefree unit that would address nicotine dependence in the context of other drug addictions. This paper reviews the process by which we accomplished that goal two years later, on July 5, 1991, and the results of this philosophical and programmatic change on the progress of the patients in their recovery.

The transition from a program which permitted (and tacitly approved of) smoking to one which prohibited smoking and addressed nicotine dependence as another drug dependency occurred in four phases: (a) making the decision to become smokefree, (b) preparing for the change, (c) implementing the change, and (d) coping with the results of the change. These phases parallel in many ways those of the transtheoretical model of change of Prochaska and DiClemente:[35] (a) moving from precontemplation to contemplation, (b) moving from contemplation to preparation, (c) moving from preparation to action, and (d) moving from action to maintenance. Viewing the transition in this way proved helpful to understanding the challenges we faced.

SUBJECTS AND METHODS

Subjects were patients in the Harris County Psychiatric Center (HCPC), a 250-bed public psychiatric hospital, staffed by faculty and residents of the Department of Psychiatry and Behavioral Sciences of the University of Texas-Houston Medical School. In 1989, two 23-bed units at HCPC (Unit 3B and Unit 3C) were devoted to the treatment of chemical dependency. The admissions department maintained a waiting list for the addiction treatment units; this list often contained the names of 50 prospective patients, and never dropped below five prospective patients during the course of this study.

On July 1, 1989, the author became Medical Director for Unit 3B, instituted a new treatment program, and announced that the unit would become smokefree in two years.

Both addiction treatment programs relied on a foundation in 12-Step recovery, although the two programs differed in the ratio of therapy groups to educational groups offered. New patients presenting to the hospital for addiction treatment were admitted to the first open bed on either Unit 3B or Unit 3C, both before and after Unit 3B became smokefree. At no time during the period of this study were patients preferentially admitted to one or the other unit; specifically, neither the smoking status of a patient or that patient's preference for a smoking or nonsmoking unit affected the unit to which the patient was admitted, and transfers from one unit to the other were not permitted. This first-open-bed policy also applied to transfers to the addictions units from elsewhere in the hospital. If a voluntary patient refused admission to either Unit 3B or Unit 3C, the bed was offered to the next patient on the waiting list. Unit 3B often admitted more than 60 patients in a month, and the admissions department never had more than three patients refuse admission or transfer to the smokefree unit in any month. Prospective patients who declined admission could place their names back on the waiting list for admission to the other unit.

Data were collected on patient admissions, discharges and degree of success in the program from July 1, 1989 through July 1, 1995. This study analyzes data on the 2458 patients admitted to Unit 3B from September 1, 1990 through July 1, 1995. Data were collected concurrently, including patient demographics (age, race, gender, legal status), progress in treatment (how much of the program the patient completed), untoward events (AWOL, AMA, seclusions, restraints), smoking status, and disposition at discharge. Data on five patients were incomplete, and these records were excluded from the analysis. Eight patients were admitted to Unit 3B in error and were immediately transferred, and these records were also excluded from the analysis. This left 2445 admissions for analysis. There were 263 admissions in Period I (September 1990-June 1991), 692 admissions in Period II (July 1991-February 1993), and 1490 admissions in Period III (March 1993-June 1995).

The independent variables in this quasi-experimental study are the program's smoking status and its requirements for program completion; the rate of program completion is the dependent variable. The two smoking status conditions (smoking permitted in Period I versus smoking not permitted in Period II and Period III) and the two length-of-stay conditions (longer length of stay in Period I and Period II and shorter length of stay in Period III) are described in detail below.

Completion of the treatment program was considered an important goal for all patients. Staff felt that those who only stayed for detoxification and those who did not complete the designated requirements had neither learned sufficient information nor developed sufficient sobriety skills to improve their chances of staying sober. Program completion was not based on length of residence in the program, but rather on completion of the following elements:

- Completion of a detailed Step I worksheet developed by the author and staff (focused on acceptance of one's addiction and understanding its consequences in one's life); presentation of this material to the group; and acceptance of the Step as being complete and sincere by the group and the group facilitator.
- Completion of a detailed Step II worksheet developed by the author and staff (focused on a consideration of one's spiritual life); presentation of this material to the group; and acceptance of the Step as being complete and sincere by the group and the group facilitator. (During Period III, the requirement for completing a Step II was dropped.)

- Completion of a detailed relapse prevention plan worksheet developed by the author and staff (focused on understanding external and internal triggers to relapse, identifying barriers to recovery, and developing strategies for dealing with these barriers); presentation of this material to the group; and acceptance of the Step as being complete and sincere by the group and the group facilitator.
- Obtaining a sponsor and three or more supporters in the AA program.
- Identifying a chemical free and appropriate living environment to go to after discharge.

The determination of "program completion" was made by a consensus of the staff, which included the nurses (who led the Step groups), the social workers (who led the relapse prevention groups), the addiction counselors (who led the education groups), and the doctors. The decision reached by staff consensus was recorded by the author at the time of discharge.

This paper does not present data on the rates at which patients maintained sobriety (from alcohol and other drugs, including nicotine) or on other outcomes following discharge. Unfortunately, the program did not have sufficient resources to follow patients after discharge beyond a limited telephone contact.

The sample included 1586 men and 859 women (65 percent to 35 percent), all medically indigent residents of Harris County (Houston), Texas. African-Americans comprised 43 percent of the sample, whites made up 46 percent, and Hispanics 11 percent. At a time when about 27 percent of American men and 24 percent of American women were smokers, 77.9 percent of the men and 78.1 percent of the women met the DSM-IIIR or DSM-IV criteria for nicotine dependence.[36,37] (DSM-IV was adopted during the course of this study.) None of the women and 4 percent of the men used smokeless tobacco in addition to cigarettes; none used smokeless tobacco exclusively. Voluntarily admitted patients comprised 61.4 percent of the sample, and involuntarily admitted patients comprised 38.6 percent; Texas law provides for involuntary commitment for chemical dependency as well as for psychiatric illnesses if the individual represents a danger to self or others. Involuntary patients were made voluntary as soon as their withdrawal symptoms had stabilized, usually within 48 hours. Previously involuntary patients who wished to remain in treatment did so; those who asked to leave were discharged within four hours of their signed request.

Data were subjected to a chi-squared analysis using SASS.

On July 1, 1989, when the author became the Medical Director of Unit

3B, smoking was permitted on the unit when groups were not in session; there was no separate smoking room. On the day he assumed leadership of Unit 3B, the author announced the goal of becoming a smokefree treatment program in the subsequent two years; the new program would not only create a smokefree environment on the unit, it would also address nicotine dependence as another chemical addiction which would be treated as part of the program. Clearing the indoor air was only one objective; the new program would not permit smoking at any time and would also provide treatment for nicotine dependence. This initiative had the support of the Department of Psychiatry and the hospital administration, although the rest of the hospital had no plans to become smokefree. (The children's unit and the two adolescent units had always been smokefree.)

During the next two years, the author and others provided extensive educational opportunities for staff in nicotine dependence and its treatment. Several staff members who were smokers took the opportunity to quit smoking; one of these staff members later became the facilitator of the nicotine dependence treatment groups.

Unit 3B was a pleasant, roomy, well-lit unit with 11 double and one single room all opening into a large, roughly triangular atrium area; only the single room (reserved for medically ill patients) had a private bathroom. Women were assigned to rooms on one side of the unit, adjacent to the women's bathroom, and men were assigned to rooms on the other side. Prior to July 1989, smoking was permitted in any of the common areas on the unit–in the atrium, outside the bathrooms, and at the telephones, though not in patient rooms, staff offices or group rooms, at all times when program activities were not in session. In January 1991, as a first effort to address nicotine dependence, the smoking area was reduced, creating a smokefree area in the main atrium; we also started an educational group on nicotine once each week, and had self-help materials that were available for all patients. In April 1991, the smoking area was again reduced in size to approximately one-fifth of the common area, and was only allowed in the areas adjacent to the men's and women's bathrooms.

On June 5, 1991, the patients on Unit 3B were informed that Unit 3B would become nonsmoking, and the times when smoking was permitted were reduced to six times daily (the patients voted on which six times). At that time, we added a nicotine dependence therapy group which was mandatory; later, this group was made voluntary. Individual counseling for nicotine dependence was available for patients who requested it; a recovery-oriented smoking cessation book was given to patients who demonstrated a commitment to recovery from nicotine dependence.[38]

On July 5, 1991 at 9:00 AM, Unit 3B became a smokefree treatment unit. All tobacco products and tobacco use paraphernalia became contraband. Patients were no longer permitted to use tobacco products on the unit or off the unit; specifically, there were no smoking breaks, and smoking was no longer permitted when attending in-house AA meetings, on outings, or during any other program activity. Consequences were introduced for possession of tobacco or lighters; shirts and hats with tobacco insignia were no longer permitted. When patients were on pass and not under staff supervision (to outside AA meetings, interviews for halfway houses, etc.) they were encouraged to refrain from smoking, but no effort was made to monitor their abstinence while they were in the community.

Nicotine polacrilex (Nicorette®) has been available since 1984; it was offered to all patients meeting the criteria for nicotine withdrawal, and most patients accepted it. Nicotine transdermal systems were approved by the Food and Drug Administration (FDA) in December 1991; Habitrol® was the first patch on the market, and it was approved by the hospital's Pharmacy and Therapeutics Committee for use within the hospital. The patch soon became the preferred method of nicotine replacement among patients.

At first, the author (and the residents) prescribed nicotine replacement products throughout the patients' hospital stays ("nicotine replacement"), but within a year, they began using nicotine replacement products in decreasing doses over several days ("nicotine detoxification"): four or five days on a 21 mg or 14 mg patch (depending on the Fagerström score[39]), reducing the dosage stepwise over one or two weeks. This detoxification strategy was as well accepted by patients as the nicotine replacement strategy had been, and afforded the patients a period of several days to several weeks time free of nicotine prior to discharge.

After going smokefree, staff incorporated nicotine dependence material in essentially every activity. For example, when explaining how addicts use chemicals to modify and control feelings, the staff member might use "alcohol, cocaine, nicotine and heroin" as examples. When describing the consequences of chemical use, a staff member might describe liver disease from alcohol, seizures from cocaine, and emphysema from smoking. Thus, staff made an effort to incorporate recovery from nicotine dependence along with recovery from other drug dependencies in all activities. In addition, attendance at the nicotine dependence therapy group was highly encouraged by all staff members.

Data for this study were collected during three distinct periods:

- Period I: When the program had more requirements (and a length of stay averaging 29 days), and was smoking permitted (September 1, 1990 through July 4, 1991).

- Period II: When the program had more requirements (and a length of stay averaging 29 days), and smoking was not permitted (July 5, 1991 though February 28, 1993).
- Period III: After the program reduced its requirements (and the length of stay averaged 17 days), and smoking was not permitted (March 1, 1993 through July 5, 1995).

RESULTS

Data collection results are displayed in Tables 1-6 and Figure 1.

Of the 2445 patients treated during the three time periods, 1124 (46 percent) completed their assigned program. No significant differences were found between the program completion rates of nicotine dependent patients ("smokers") and those who did not meet the criteria for nicotine dependence ("nonsmokers"), or between the program completion rates of men and women, or of any ethnic group. Not surprisingly, involuntary patients chose to leave treatment before completing the program more often than voluntary patients; overall, 59.1 percent of voluntary patients and 25.0 percent of involuntary patients completed the program (p = .001). Smoking status did not affect involuntary patients' decisions to stay or leave; the program completion rates for involuntary smokers and involuntary nonsmokers were similar, as were the program completion rates for voluntary smokers and voluntary nonsmokers.

Women nonsmokers had a higher overall rate of program completion than men nonsmokers and all smokers (p < .001), and in each of the three periods: 66.7 percent in the first period, 51.1 percent in the second period, and 61.4 percent in the third period (differences between women non-smokers and others, significant p = .001).

The average rates of program completion during each of the three time periods show overall consistency. When smoking was permitted and the longer program was required (Period I), 49.4 percent of patients completed the program; after smoking was no longer permitted (Period II), 44.7 percent of the patients completed the program; and after the required program was reduced and smoking was still not permitted (Period III), 46 percent of the patients completed the program (differences not significant). The program completion rates across the three time periods among men, women, all ethnic groups, smokers and nonsmokers were also similar (and did not show a statistically significant difference).

An analysis of the transition period from smoking to nonsmoking yielded additional information. In the three-month period immediately following this transition (July, August and September, 1991), the program

TABLE 1. Summary of demographics.

Patients admitted:	2458	
Records dropped from analysis:	13	
Records analyzed:	2445	
Ethnicity		
African-American	1051	(43.0%)
White	1121	(45.8%)
Hispanic	260	(10.6%)
Other	13	(<1%)
Gender:		
Women	859	(35.1%)
Men	1586	(64.9%)
Legal status		
Voluntary	1501	(61.4%)
Involuntary	944	(38.6%)
Nicotine dependence status at admission:		
Met criteria ("smokers")	1907	(78.0%)
Did not meet criteria ("nonsmokers")	538	(22.0%)
Program completion:		
Completed the program	1124	(46.0%)
Did not complete the program	1321	(54.0%)

TABLE 2. Patients who met or did not meet the criteria for nicotine dependence 305.10. 2445 consecutive admissions to an inpatient addiction treatment program.

	Met criteria for nicotine dependence (%) ("smokers")	Did not meet criteria for nicotine dependence (%) ("nonsmokers")	All patients
Men	1236 (77.9)	350 (22.1)	1586
Women	671 (78.1)	188 (21.9)	859
All patients	1907 (78.0)	538 (22.0)	2445

Percentages are shown in parentheses.

completion rate declined precipitously from 49.4 percent to 30.7 percent; there were no differences related to gender or ethnic group. More importantly, the program completion rate for nonsmokers declined to the same degree as that of smokers after the unit became smokefree. Three months later, however, the program completion rate had returned to the level seen

TABLE 3. Patients who completed the designated addiction treatment program, nicotine dependence status. 2445 consecutive admissions to an inpatient addiction treatment program.

	Met criteria for nicotine dependence (%) ("smokers")		Did not meet criteria for nicotine dependence (%) ("nonsmokers")		All patients	
	Completed (%)	Total	Completed (%)	Total	Completed (%)	Total
Men	564 (45.6)	1236	164 (46.9)	350	728 (45.9)	1586
Women	285 (42.5)	671	111 (59.0)*	188	396 (46.1)	859
All patients	849 (44.5)	1907	275 (51.1)	538	1124 (46.0)	2445

Percentages are shown in parentheses.

* Women nonsmokers had a higher rate of program completion than women nonsmokers and all smokers (p < .001).

TABLE 4. Program completion rates, before and after the program became smokefree, and after it reduced its length of stay.

		Period I: Smoking permitted, long LOS		Period II: Smoking prohibited, long LOS		Period III: Smoking prohibited, short LOS	
		Completed (%)	All patients	Completed (%)	All patients	Completed (%)	All patients
Men +ND	AA	37 (55.2)	67	79 (49.1)	161	148 (51.2)	289
	W	26 (39.4)	66	79 (47.0)	168	151 (43.2)	349
	H	6 (46.2)	13	12 (28.6)	42	24 (32.9)	73
	O	0	0	0 (00.0)	2	2 (33.3)	6
	All	69 (47.2)	146	170 (45.6)	373	325 (45.3)	717
Women +ND	AA	15 (39.5)	38	35 (40.7)	86	71 (42.8)	166
	W	27 (56.2)	48	39 (39.4)	99	80 (41.5)	193
	H	2 (40.0)	5	9 (56.2)	16	7 (41.2)	17
	O	0	0	0	0	0 (0.00)	3
	All	44 (48.4)	91	83 (41.3)	201	158 (41.7)	379
Men −ND	AA	4 (80.0)	5	21 (61.8)	34	60 (50.0)	120
	W	3 (42.9)	7	8 (34.8)	23	39 (46.4)	84
	H	4 (80.0)	5	3 (21.4)	14	22 (38.0)	58
	O	0	0	0	0	0	0
	All	11 (64.7)	17	32 (45.1)	71	121 (46.2)	262

Women	AA	2 (40.0)	5	10 (58.9)	17	41 (65.1)	63
-ND	W	4 (100.0)	4	9 (37.5)	24	35 (62.5)	56
	H	0	0	4 (80.0)	5	4 (33.3)	12
	O	0	0	1 (100.0)	1	1 (1.000)	1
	All	6 (66.7)*	9	24 (51.1)*	47	81 (61.4)*	132
All Men		80 (49.1)	163	202 (45.5)	444	446 (45.6)	979
All Women		50 (50.0)	100	107 (43.1)	248	239 (46.8)	511
All +ND		113 (47.7)	237	253 (44.1)	574	483 (44.1)	1096
All -ND		17 (65.4)	26	56 (47.5)	118	202 (51.3)	394
All patients		130 (49.4)	263	309 (44.7)	692	685 (46.0)	1490

Period I: September 1, 1990-July 4, 1991
Period II: July 5, 1991-February 28, 1993
Period III: March 1, 1993-July 5, 1995

AA   African-American
W   White
H   Hispanic
O   Other
+ND Met the criteria for nicotine dependence ("smokers")
-ND Did not meet the criteria for nicotine dependence ("nonsmokers")

Percentages are shown in parentheses.

* Women nonsmokers had a higher rate of program completion than women nonsmokers and all smokers (p < .001) in all three periods. Other differences were not statistically significant.

TABLE 5. Patients who completed the program after it became smokefree, based on their nicotine dependence status. 692 consecutive admissions to a smokefree inpatient addiction treatment program.

	First 3 months		Middle 14 months		Last 3 months		All patients
	Completed (%)	All	Completed (%)	All	Completed (%)	All	
+ND ("smokers")	23 (30.7)	75	167 (41.7)	401	63 (64.3)	98	574
−ND ("nonsmokers")	4 (30.8)	13	44 (49.4)	89	8 (50.0)	16	118
All patients	27 (30.7)	88	211 (43.1)	490	71 (62.3)	114	692

+ND   Met the criteria for nicotine dependence
−ND   Did not meet the criteria for nicotine dependence

Percentages are shown in parentheses.

* Differences between first 3 months, middle 14 months, and last 3 months are significant, $p = .001$, for smokers, nonsmokers, and for all patients. Differences between smokers and nonsmokers are not statistically significant.

TABLE 6. Patients who completed the designated addiction treatment program, by legal status and nicotine dependence status. 2445 consecutive admissions to an inpatient addiction treatment program.

	Met criteria for nicotine dependence (%) ("smokers")		Did not meet criteria for nicotine dependence (%) ("nonsmokers")		All patients	
	Completed (%)	Total	Completed (%)	Total	Completed (%)	Total
Voluntary admission	664 (57.9)	1147	224 (63.3)	354	888 (59.1)	1501
Involuntary admission	185 (24.3)	760	51 (27.7)*	184	236 (25.0)	944
All patients	849 (44.5)	1907	275 (51.1)	538	1124 (46.0)	2445

Percentages are shown in parentheses.

* Differences between voluntary smokers and involuntary smokers are significant (p < .001).
* Differences between voluntary smokers and involuntary nonsmokers are significant (p < .001).
* Differences between voluntary smokers and nonsmokers, and between involuntary smokers and nonsmokers, are not significant.

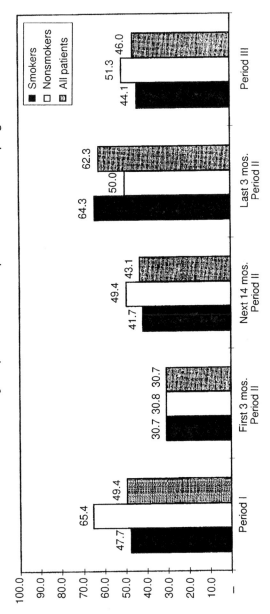

FIGURE 1. Percentage of patients who completed the treatment program.

before the program went smokefree (for both smokers and nonsmokers), and the program completion rate for the following 14 months averaged 43.1 percent. After being smokefree for 17 months, the program completion rate was even higher (again, for both smokers and nonsmokers); the program completion rate for December 1992, January and February 1993 (the last three months of this period) was 62.3 percent. (The differences between time periods were statistically significant [p = .001]). This pattern—a drop in the program completion rate following the transition with a return to baseline in three months and subsequent further improvement—was evident for both smokers and nonsmokers (64.3 percent for smokers and 50.0 percent for nonsmokers, difference not statistically significant).

When averaged across each time period, the program completion rate of nonsmokers did not improve and the program completion rate for smokers did not worsen after going smokefree (except during the transition period, when the rate for both groups declined by about the same amount).

In addition to collecting program completion data, we also monitored untoward events in the milieu, including restraints, seclusions, "codes," and aggressive behavior by patients toward staff, peers, and inanimate objects. These events were extremely rare both before and after becoming smokefree; the seclusion room was used about twice a year. There were no changes in the rates of occurrence of such events during the three periods. We also monitored AWOLs, and administrative discharges for rules violations; there were no changes in the rates of these untoward events during the three periods.

DISCUSSION

The similarity in program completion rates across time periods ran counter to our expectations and the fears of the hospital's administration; we had anticipated that nonsmokers would prefer a nonsmoking environment and would be more likely to complete treatment after the unit became smokefree. Similarly, we expected the program completion rate of smokers to decline after going smokefree, due to the increased stress of nicotine withdrawal and the limitation of personal freedom from interdiction of tobacco. Neither event occurred. The data reveal that, following the disruptive transition period, the program completion rates of both smokers and nonsmokers returned to previous levels after the unit became smokefree.

The rate of program completion dropped significantly during the three months immediately after the unit became smokefree. However, the content of the treatment program itself did not change significantly during these three months–we had begun providing nicotine dependence programming five months earlier. Neither the admitting procedures nor the types of patients admitted changed, and there was no staff turnover. The only major changes were the rules regarding tobacco use. One might conclude that the patients did not like the new rules and left prematurely so they could smoke. The data, however, do not support this conclusion:

- The program completion rate for nonsmokers dropped just as steeply as the rate for smokers after becoming smokefree.
- Three months after becoming smokefree, the program completion rate for both smokers and nonsmokers returned to the levels seen before making the change.
- After seventeen months, the program completion rates were significantly higher yet, for both smokers and nonsmokers (and the completion rate for smokers was actually higher than that of nonsmokers).

We concluded that the reason for the drop in program completion rates after becoming smokefree was due to the disruption to the established program, independent of the reason for the disruption. Programmatic change–any change–creates stress among both staff and patients, which interferes in the ability of the staff to provide services and of the patients to utilize them. After becoming a smokefree unit, some staff members were uncertain about their new roles and responsibilities, and some disagreed with the policy change altogether. Some wanted to enforce the rules aggressively and others wanted to be more forgiving, leading to uncertainty in the milieu. In addition, although most staff members who previously smoked had quit smoking by the time the unit became smokefree, five staff members were still smokers (two nurses and three technicians). These staff members were understandably ambivalent about supporting the new policy.

Individuals who were inpatients at the time of the transition (July 5, 1991) experienced a significant programmatic change–suddenly, the milieu was focused on smoking instead of the process of addiction recovery. Patients admitted during the ensuing month did not experience the transition, but were with peers who had. By August 1991, none of the current patients had been in the program when smoking was permitted, and as time passed, the recollection of a unit with a smoking milieu became a more and more distant memory.

Three months after going smokefree, most staff members had accepted the change as permanent and had developed more effective approaches to deal with patient discontent; we became more consistent in stating and enforcing policies and developed better nicotine dependence programming. As the staff stabilized, the patient milieu adjusted to being smokefree. This improved stability was reflected in an improved program completion rate.

The experience of Unit 3B suggests that a minimum of three average-length-of-stay cycles are required before the milieu returns to stability:

- Patients who had witnessed the transition said "We used to be able to smoke on the unit–why can't we smoke now?" and felt bitter.
- Patients who were admitted after the transition but who interacted with other patients who did witness the transition said "I've heard that they used to be able to smoke on the unit–why can't we smoke now?" and felt resentful.
- Patients who were admitted sufficiently long after the transition that they did not come into contact with patients who had personally witnessed the transition, but who had heard about the transition second-hand, said "I heard how they used to be able to smoke on the unit–why can't we?" and felt angry.
- Eventually, no patients even knew patients who knew patients who had witnessed the transition. At that point, the concept of smoking on the unit passed into folklore, and patients simply said "Why can't we smoke on the unit?" and felt disappointed.

Patients' unhappiness at not being allowed to smoke during treatment (after the transition period) did not prove to be a major barrier. Typically, the attending physician or resident would meet the patient in the admitting office prior to admission and discuss the smokefree status of the unit. Prospective patients read the policy on tobacco use and signed a statement acknowledging and accepting the rules. The vast majority of patients were in Contemplation stage, making statements such as, "I need to quit smoking anyway," and "I might as well quit everything."

Even though patients accepted the smokefree policy in theory, many (perhaps most) violated the policy on occasion. We monitored these events as carefully as possible. During Period I, smoking was permitted and cigarettes could be freely brought onto the unit. During Periods II and III, some patients smuggled cigarettes onto the unit from time to time. After considerable thought and some experimentation, the treatment team settled on the following consequences for violations of the smoking/tobacco rules:

- First violation: Restriction from the cafeteria for 24 hours (patients ate alone on the unit and missed the social interaction of mealtime).
- Second violation: Restriction from the cafeteria for 48 hours.
- Third violation: Administrative dismissal.

We dismissed about one patient each month during the first few months of the smokefree period, and discovered that more careful attention to the milieu reduced the number of cigarettes smuggled onto the unit. When we did occasional room searches and cursory personal searches, the patients attempted to bring cigarettes onto the unit quite frequently, and the aroma of cigarette smoke filled the bathrooms every day. When we instituted daily room searches as a matter of course, the amount of smoking greatly decreased. Toward the end of the study period, no more than one patient was dismissed for tobacco rules violations every three months.

As the staff got better at searching and clearer about their responsibilities, the patients became more clever at hiding cigarettes. At first, staff found cigarettes in drawers and on shelves; later, only in pockets and under mattresses; then, between pages of books and in the toes of dirty socks. Some patients became extremely resourceful, hiding cigarettes in the hem of the drapes, inside a toilet paper roll, and behind a loose tile in the bathroom. In parallel, the price of smuggled cigarettes increased, eventually reaching one dollar per cigarette (or so we were told).

The fact that some patients went to great lengths to smuggle, hide, sell and smoke cigarettes in violation of the rules indicated several things:

- Sneaking and smoking a single cigarette (and risking dismissal by doing so) could not be explained on the basis on nicotine withdrawal, since nicotine patches and nicotine polacrilex were freely available. It is more easily explained as acting-out behavior or as addictive behavior ("a dope-fiend move," in local slang) and confronting it as such proved more effective than treating it as a plea for more nicotine replacement.
- While some patients were vehemently opposed to the smokefree policy, most chose to stay in treatment in spite of it.
- Violations of the smoking/tobacco policies were usually seen in conjunction with other rules violations (such as curfew violations, inappropriate interpersonal touching, going into other patients' rooms, and hoarding food).
- Once reprimanded and redirected, most patients followed the rules.

Relatively few addiction treatment programs were smokefree in 1989 when Unit 3B began this process.[40,41] Since then, however, essentially all treatment programs have cleared the indoor air of tobacco smoke, and many have integrated nicotine dependence treatment into their programs. Published reports of these initiatives indicate varying degrees of success, but overall they demonstrate, as we did, that incorporating nicotine dependence into the context of addiction treatment and psychiatric treatment is feasible, viable, and advantageous to patients.[42-63]

This study followed the course of medically indigent patients in Houston, Texas, who were treated in a publicly-funded, university-based treatment center. Other treatment settings with dissimilar patients may find different results. Specifically, having one physician responsible for the care of all patients allowed us to maintain consistent unit policies; units with many attending physicians might find this more difficult. Also, our patients had few other options regarding treatment; privately-insured patients might be more reluctant to accept a smokefree treatment center. However, private treatment centers might also expect a higher overall level of program completion; our patients' limited resources and low socioeconomic status represented serious barriers to recovery, and the involuntary patients (less commonly seen in private settings) had a lower program completion rate than the voluntary patients.

The treatment unit under study accepted both voluntary and involuntary patients; involuntary patients were made voluntary as soon as their detoxification was stabilized, usually within 48 hours. We were pleased that a substantial percentage of these patients applied themselves to the program and completed it (25.0 percent overall). There did not appear to be an interaction between legal status and smoking status with regard to program completion; a similar percentage of involuntarily admitted smokers and nonsmokers completed the program (24.3 percent and 27.7 percent, respectively), and this was true in all three time periods.

We did not evaluate the effects of this program on abstinence rates or other measures of program success, and we did not evaluate the effectiveness of the program in helping patients quit smoking, because the hospital did not have the financial resources to complete an outcome study.

CONCLUSIONS

These data demonstrate that the disruption caused by becoming a smoke-free addiction treatment unit stabilized after three months, and that the ability of patients (both smokers and nonsmokers) to complete the program then returned to baseline levels. The fears that large numbers of patients would refuse to be admitted or would leave prematurely, and the concerns that staff would not be equal to the task, proved to be unfounded.

This brief report does not fully communicate either the satisfaction or the pride felt by the author and the Unit 3B staff in succeeding in this endeavor. Nor does it reflect the frustrations and acrimonious dissension that occasionally peppered staff interactions many times during these six years. Becoming a smokefree treatment unit stressed everyone's ability to stay focused on progress and recovery (of the patients, of the staff, and of the treatment unit); steadfast dedication to principles and a willingness to compromise proved to be essential to success.

Our experience can be summarized into a few suggestions for other programs seeking to make the transition to a smokefree program; more detailed information can obtained from the Addressing Tobacco in the Treatment of Other Addictions Project in New Brunswick, NJ:[59]

- Start at the top; unless the CEO supports the policy, it will fail.
- Agree on goals: how smokefree will you be?
- Agree on a reasonable timetable for change that takes into account the existing culture, sources of support, and the current stage of change of the staff and the institution.[64]
- Plan carefully, then educate widely; educate *all* staff, but a few staff members must become expert in order to lead the groups and provide individual counseling.
- Establish policies and procedures, and be certain everyone is familiar with them.
- Encourage and nurture cooperation from every source (security, housekeeping, maintenance, dietary, admissions).
- Staff who still smoke must not be identifiable as smokers by the patients.
- Initiate treatment modalities in advance of the policy change.
- Move swiftly from smoking to smokefree; a slow transition prolongs the pain.
- Expect programmatic disruption for a minimum of three patient cycles.
- Utilize the experience of others, through formal and informal consultations, written materials, workbooks and films.
- Enforce the rules for the benefit of the milieu.
- Do not expect gratitude from patients, their families, staff, or administrators; very few will recognize that progress is often painful.
- Take pride in the policy; tobacco kills more than 400,000 Americans every year, and more alcoholics die tobacco-related deaths than alcohol-related deaths.[65]
- Be patient; paradigm shifts are never easy.

The author concurs with the Agency for Health Care Policy and Research[66] and with the American Society of Addiction Medicine[67] that nicotine dependence treatment belongs in the mainstream of medical and addiction treatment. The data presented here support the argument that addiction treatment programs can institute a tobacco-free policy and incorporate nicotine dependence treatment into the context of their programs without adversely affecting the progress of the patients through treatment. These data also suggest that the disruption caused by going smokefree has more to do with resistance to change than resistance to dealing with nicotine dependence.

REFERENCES

1. Benowitz NL. Drug Therapy: Pharmacologic aspects of cigarette smoking and nicotine addiction. N Engl J Med 1988; 319:1318-1330.

2. Cohen C, Pickworth WB, Henningfield JE. Cigarette smoking and addiction. Clin Chest Med 1991; 12:701-710.

3. Henningfield JE, Cohen C, Slade JD. Is nicotine more addicting than cocaine? Brit J Addict 1991; 86:565-569.

4. Henningfield JE, Miyasato K, Jasinski DR. Abuse liability and pharmacodynamic characteristics of intravenous and inhaled nicotine. J Pharmacol Exp Ther 1985;234:1-12.

5. Battjes RJ. Smoking as an issue in alcohol and drug abuse treatment. Addict Behav 1988;13:225-230.

6. U.S. Department of Health and Human Services. The Health Consequences of Smoking: Nicotine Addiction. Rockville, MD: U.S. Department of Health and Human Services, Public Health Service, Office on Smoking and Health, DHHS Publication 88-8406, 1988.

7. Breslau N. Psychiatric comorbidity of smoking and nicotine dependence. Behav Genet 1995;25(2):95-101.

8. Breslau N, Kilbey MM, Andreski P. Vulnerability to psychopathology in nicotine-dependent smokers: an epidemiologic study of young adults. Am J Psychiatry 1993;150(6):941-946.

9. Gulliver SB, Rohsenow DJ, Colby SM, Dey AN, Abrams DB, Niaura RS, Monti PM. Interrelationship of smoking and alcohol dependence, use and urges to use. J Stud Alcohol 1995;56(2):202-206.

10. Kozlowski LT, Henningfield JE, Keenan RM, Lei H, Leigh G, Jelinek LC, Pope MA, Haertzen CA. Patterns of alcohol, cigarette, and caffeine and other drug use in two drug abusing populations. J Subst Abuse Treat 1993;10(2):171-179.

11. Lerman C, Audrain J, Orleans CT, Boyd R, Gold K, Main D, Caporaso N. Investigation of mechanisms linking depressed mood to nicotine dependence. Addict Behav 1996;21(1):9-19.

12. Murray RP, Istvan JA, Voelker HT, Rigdon MA, Wallace MD. Level of involvement with alcohol and success at smoking cessation in the lung health study. J Stud Alcohol 1995;56(1):74-82.

13. Nisell M, Nomikos GG, Svensson TH. Nicotine dependence, midbrain dopamine systems and psychiatric disorders. Pharmacol Toxicol 1995;76(3):157-162.

14. Ochoa EL. Nicotine-related brain disorders: the neurobiological basis of nicotine dependence. Cell Mol Neurobiol 1994;14(3):195-225.

15. Stark MJ, Campbell BK. Drug use and cigarette smoking in applicants for drug abuse treatment. J Subst Abuse 1993;5(2):175-181.

16. Knapp JM, Kottke TE, Heitzig C. A controlled trial to implement smoke-free hospitals. Minn Med 1989;72:713-716.

17. Knapp JM, Rosheim CL, Meister EA, Kottke TE. Managing tobacco dependence in chemical dependency treatment facilities: a survey of current attitudes and policies. J Addict Dis 1993;12(4):89-104.

18. Kottke TE. The smoke-free hospital: A smoke-free worksite. NY State J Med. 1989;89:38-42.

19. Bobo JK. Nicotine dependence and alcoholism: Epidemiology and treatment. J Psychoactive Drugs 1989;21(3):323-329.

20. Bobo JK, Davis CM. Recovering staff and smoking in chemical dependency programs in rural Nebraska. J Subst Abuse Treat 1993;10:221-228.

21. Catford JC, Nutbeam D. Smoking in hospitals. Lancet 1983;2:94-96.

22. Dingman P, Resnick M, Bosworth E, Kamada D. A nonsmoking policy on an acute psychiatric unit. Journal of Psychosocial Nursing and Mental Health Services 1988;26:11-14.

23. Erwin S, Biordi D. A smoke-free environment: Psychiatric nurses respond. Journal of Psychosocial Nursing and Mental Health Services 1991;29:12-18.

24. Goldsmith RJ, Hurt RD, Slade J. The development of smoke-free chemical dependency units. J Addict Dis 1991;11:67-77.

25. Resnick MP, Bosworth EE. A smoke-free psychiatric unit. Hosp Comm Psychiatry. 1989;40:525-527.

26. Resnick M, Gordon R, Bosworth EE. Evolution of smoking policies in Oregon psychiatric facilities. Hosp Comm Psychiatry. 1989;40:527-529.

27. Smith WR, Grant BL. Effects of a smoking ban on general hospital psychiatric service. Hosp Comm Psychiatry. 1989;40:497-502.

28. Delaney GO. Tobacco dependence in treating alcoholism. NJ Med 1988; 85:131-132.

29. Pletcher VC. Nicotine treatment at the Drug Dependency Program of the Minneapolis VA Medical Center: A program director's perspective. J Subst Abuse Treat 1993:10:1139-1146.

30. Dawley HH. Toward a smoke-free VA. VA Practitioner 1989;4:47-65.

31. Gritz ER, Stapleton JM, Hill MA, Jana ME. Prevalence of cigarette smoking in VA medical and psychiatric hospitals. Bulletin of the Society of Psychologists on Addictive Behaviors 1985;4:151-165.

32. Capretto NA. Confronting nicotine dependency at the Gateway Rehabilitation Center. J Subst Abuse Treat 1993;10:113-116.

33. Karan LD. Initial encounters with tobacco cessation on the Inpatient Substance Abuse Unit of the Medical College of Virginia. J Subst Abuse Treat 1993;10:117-124.

34. Hurt RD, Dale LC, McClain FL, Eberman KM, Offord KP, Bruce BK, Lauger GG. A comprehensive model for the treatment of nicotine dependence in a medical setting. Med Clin North America 1992;76:495-514.

35. Prochaska JO, DiClemente CC. Toward a comprehensive model of change. In: Miller WR, Hester NK, eds. Treating addictive behaviors: Processes of change. New York: Plenum Press, 1986:3-27.

36. American Psychiatric Association. Diagnostic and Statistical Manual of Mental Disorders, Third Edition, Revised. New York: APA Press, 1987.

37. American Psychiatric Association. Diagnostic and Statistical Manual of Mental Disorders, Fourth Edition. New York: APA Press, 1994.

38. Rustin TA. Quit and Stay Quit: A personal program to stop smoking. Center City, MN: Hazelden Educational Materials, 1991.

39. Heatherton TF, Kozlowski LT, Frecker RC, Fagerström KO. The Fagerstrom Test for Nicotine Dependence: A revision of the Fagerstrom Tolerance Questionnaire. Brit J Addict 1991;86:1119-1127.

40. Goldsmith RJ, Knapp J. Towards a broader view of recovery. J Subst Abuse Treat 1993;10(2):107-111.

41. Hoffman AL, Slade J. Following the pioneers: Addressing tobacco in chemical dependency treatment. J Subst Abuse Treat 1993;10(2):153-160.

42. Bernstein SM, Madonik B, Schwalb J, Hoskins G. Effects of introducing a choice-based program for smoking at an abstinence-based treatment center. J Addict Dis 1996;15:148.

43. Bobo JK, Slade J, Hoffman AL. Nicotine addiction counseling for chemically dependent patients. Psychiatr Serv 1995;46(9):945-947.

44. Campbell BK, Wander N, Stark MI, Holbert T. Treating cigarette smoking in drug-abusing clients. J Subst Abuse Treat 1995;12(2):89-94.

45. Haller E, McNiel DE, Binder RL. Impact of a smoking ban on a locked psychiatric unit. J Clin Psychiatry 1996;57(8):329-332.

46. Hughes JR. Treatment of smoking cessation in smokers with past alcohol/drug problems. J Subst Abuse Treat 1993;10(2):181-187.

47. Hurt RD, Croghan IT, Offord KP, Eberman KM, Morse RM. Attitudes toward nicotine dependence among chemical dependence unit staff–before and after a smoking cessation trial. J Subst Abuse Treat 1995;12(4):247-252.

48. Hurt RD, Dale LC. Inpatient treatment of severe nicotine dependence. Mayo Clin Proc 1992;67:823-828.

49. Hurt RD, Dale LC, Offord KP, Croghan IT, Hays JT, Gomez-Dahl L. Nicotine patch therapy for smoking cessation in recovering alcoholics. Addiction 1995;90(11):1541-1546.

50. Hurt RD, Eberman KM, Croghan IT, Offord KP, Davis LJ Jr, Morse RM, Palmen MA, Bruce BK. Nicotine dependence treatment during inpatient treatment for other addictions: a prospective intervention trial. Alcohol Clin Exp Res 1994;18(4):867-872.

51. Joseph AM. Nicotine treatment at the Drug Dependency Program of the Minneapolis VA Medical Center. A researcher's perspective. J Subst Abuse Treat 1993;10(2):147-152.

52. Joseph AM, Nichol KL, Anderson H. Effect of treatment for nicotine dependence on alcohol and drug treatment outcomes. Addict Behav 1993;18(6):635-644.

53. Kempf J, Stanley A. Impact of tobacco-free policy on recruitment and retention of adolescents in residential substance abuse treatment. J Addict Dis 1996;15(2):1-11.

54. Ker M, Leischow S, Markowitz IB, Merikle E. Involuntary smoking cessation: a treatment option in chemical dependency programs for women and children. J Psychoactive Drugs 1996;28(1):47-60.

55. Kottke TE, Battista RN, DeFriese GH, Brekke ML. Attributes of successful smoking cessation interventions in medical practice: A meta-analysis of 39 controlled trials. JAMA 1988;259:2883-2889.

56. Kotz MM. A smoke-free chemical dependency unit. The Cleveland Clinic experience. J Subst Abuse Treat 1993;10(2):125-131.

57. Orleans CT, Hutchinson D. Tailoring nicotine addiction treatments for chemical dependency patients. J Subst Abuse Treat 1993;10(2):197-208.

58. Sees KL, Clark HW. When to begin smoking cessation in substance abusers. J Subst Abuse Treat 1993;10(2):189-195.

59. Slade J, Hoffman AL. Addressing tobacco in the treatment of other addictions: Steps for becoming tobacco-free. New Brunswick, NJ: Addressing Tobacco in the Treatment of Other Addictions, 1992.

60. Toneatto A, Sobell LC, Sobell MB, Kozlowski LT. Effect of cigarette smoking on alcohol treatment outcome. J Subst Abuse 1995;7(2):245-252.

61. Trudeau DL, Isenhart C, Silversmith D. Efficacy of smoking cessation strategies in a treatment program. J Addict Dis 1995;14(1):109-116.

62. Henningfield JE, Clayton R, Pollin W. Involvement of tobacco in alcoholism and illicit drug use. Brit J Addict 1990;85(2):279-291.

63. Joseph AM, Nichol KL, Willenbring ML, Korn JE, Lysaght LS. Beneficial effects of treatment of nicotine dependence during an inpatient substance abuse treatment program. JAMA 1990;263(22):3043-3046.

64. DiClemente CC, Prochaska JO, Fairhurst SK, Velicer WF, Velasquez MM, Rossi JS. The process of smoking cessation: An analysis of precontemplation, contemplation, and preparation stages of change. J Consult Clin Psychology 1991;59:295-304.

65. Hurt RD, Offord KP, Croghan IT, Gomez-Dahl L, Kottke TE, Morse RM, Melton LJ 3rd. Mortality following inpatient addictions treatment. Role of tobacco use in a community-based cohort. JAMA 1996;275(14):1097-1103.

66. The Agency for Health Care Policy and Research. Smoking Cessation Clinical Practice Guidelines. JAMA 1996;275(16):1270-1280.

67. American Society of Addiction Medicine. Public policy statement on nicotine dependence and tobacco. 1997; http://www.asam.org

SELECTIVE GUIDE TO CURRENT REFERENCE SOURCES ON TOPICS DISCUSSED IN THIS ISSUE

Lynn Kasner Morgan, MLS

Each issue of *Journal of Addictive Diseases* features a section offering suggestions on where to look for further information on included topics. The intent is to guide readers to selective substantive sources of current information.

Some published reference works utilize designated terminology (controlled vocabularies) which must be used to find material on topics of interest. For these, a sample of available search terms has been indicated to assist the reader in accessing appropriate sources for his/her purposes. Other reference tools use keywords or free text terms from the title of the document, the abstract, and the name of any responsible agency or conference. In searching using keywords, be sure to look under all possible synonyms to retrieve the concept in question.

Lynn Kasner Morgan is Assistant Professor of Medical Education, Assistant Dean for Information Resources and Systems, and Director of the Gustave L. and Janet W. Levy Library of the Mount Sinai Medical Center, Inc., One Gustave L. Levy Place, New York, NY 10029-6574.

[Haworth co-indexing entry note]: "Selective Guide to Current Reference Sources on Topics Discussed in This Issue." Morgan, Lynn Kasner. Co-published simultaneously in *Journal of Addictive Diseases* (The Haworth Medical Press, an imprint of The Haworth Press, Inc.) Vol. 17, No. 1, 1998, pp. 109-121; and: *Smoking and Illicit Drug Use* (ed: Mark S. Gold, and Barry Stimmel) The Haworth Medical Press, an imprint of The Haworth Press, Inc., 1998, pp. 109-121. Single or multiple copies of this article are available for a fee from The Haworth Document Delivery Service [1-800-342-9678, 9:00 a.m. - 5:00 p.m. (EST). E-mail address: getinfo@haworth.com].

An asterisk (*) appearing before a published source indicates that all or part of that source is in machine-readable form and can be accessed through an online database search. Database searching is recommended for retrieving sources of information that coordinate multiple variables, concepts, or subject areas. Most libraries offer database services which can include mediated online searching, access to locally mounted datafiles, front-end software packages, CD-ROM technology and access to the World Wide Web. Searching can also be done from one's office or home with subscriptions to database service vendors and microcomputers equipped with modems.

Interactive electronic communications systems, such as electronic mail, discussion groups, bulletin boards, and receiving and transferring files are available through the Internet, which offers timely and global information resources in all disciplines, including the health sciences. Some groups which might be of interest are: ALCOHOL (ALCOHOL@LMUACAD), DRUG ABUSE (DRUGABUS@UMAB), 12STEP@TRWRB.DSD.COM and ADDICTION MEDICINE (MAJORDOMO@AVOCADO.PC.HELSINKI.FI). The National Clearinghouse for Alcohol and Drug Information Center for Substance Abuse Prevention maintains PREVLINE, a bulletin board for alcohol and drug information. Information from PREVLINE is available through the Internet at www.health.org and a recent search included such things as results of the 1995 National Household Survey on Drug Abuse. There are also many sites with World Wide Web pages which can be reached by individuals with a Web browser such as Microsoft Explorer or Netscape. Netscape "net search" allows searching with many different web search engines. Suggested starting points are http://www.yahoo.com/health, Web Crawler searching tool http://webcrawler.com or World Wide Web Worm http://wwwmcb.cs.colorado.edu/home/mcbryan/wwww.html. Other sites to try include: Web of Addictions at http://www.well.com/user/woa; American Psychological Association Division of Pharmacology and Substance Abuse at http://charlotte.med.nyu.edu/woodr/div28.html; and Online AA resources at http://www.recovery.org. The National Information Services Corporation has made Tobacco and Health Abstracts available on the Web for a fee at http://www.nisc.com. The amount of information available on the Internet increases daily and attention should be given to the author/provider of the information which ranges from highly respected institutions to individuals with a home computer and a desire to "publish."

Readers are encouraged to consult their librarians for further assistance before undertaking research on a topic.

Suggestions regarding the content and organization of this section are welcome and should be sent to the author.

1. INDEXING AND ABSTRACTING SOURCES

Place of publication, publisher, start date, frequency of publication, and brief descriptions are noted.

Biological Abstracts (1926-) and *Biological Abstracts/RRM* (v.18, 1980-). Philadelphia, BioSciences Information Service, semimonthly. Reports on worldwide research in the life sciences.

> See: Concept headings for abstracts, such as behavioral biology, pharmacology, psychiatry, public health, and toxicology sections.

> See: Keyword-in-context subject index.

> See Also: http://www.biosis.org

Chemical Abstracts. Columbus, Ohio, American Chemical Society, 1907- , weekly. A key to the world's literature of chemistry and chemical engineering, including serial publications, proceedings and edited collections, technical reports, dissertations, new book and audiovisual materials announcements, and patent documents.

> See: *Index Guide* for cross-referencing and indexing policies.

> See: *General Subject Index* terms, such as drug dependence, drug-drug interactions, drug tolerance.

> See: Keyword subject indexes.

> See Also: http://info.cas.org

Dissertation Abstracts International. Section A. The Humanities and Social Sciences and Section B. The Sciences and Engineering. Ann Arbor, MI, University Microfilms, v.30, 1969/70- , monthly. Includes author-prepared abstracts of doctoral dissertations from 500 participating institutions throughout North America and the world. A separate section contains European dissertations.

> See: Keyword subject index.

> See Also: http://www.umi.com/hp/Products/Dissertations.html

Excerpta Medica. Amsterdam, The Netherlands, Excerpta Medica Foundation, 1947- , 42 subject sections.

A major abstracting service covering more than 4,300 biomedical journals. The abstracts, including English summaries for non-English-language articles, appear in one or more of the published subject sections, excluding Section 38, *Adverse Reactions Titles,* which is an index only. Each of the sections has a comprehensive subject index. Since 1978 all the *Excerpta Medica* sections have been available for computer searching in the integrated online file, EMBASE. Particularly relevant to the topics in this issue are Section 40, *Drug Dependence, Alcohol Abuse and Alcoholism*; and the sections that have addiction, alcoholism, or drug subdivisions: Section 30, *Clinical and Experimental Pharmacology*; Section 32, *Psychiatry*; and Section 17, *Public Health, Social Medicine and Epidemiology.*

See Also: http://www.excerptamedica.nl

Hospital and Health Administration Index. Chicago, American Hospital Association, v.51, 1995- , three issues per year, with annual cumulations. Published as the primary guide to literature on the organization and administration of hospitals and other healthcare providers, the financing and delivery of healthcare, the development and implementation of health policy and reform, and health planning and research.

See: *MeSH* terms, such as alcoholism; caffeine; comorbidity; depression; metabolic detoxication, drug; naltrexone; nicotine; substance abuse; substance abuse detection; substance abuse treatment centers; substance dependence; substance withdrawal syndrome; tobacco; tobacco use disorder.

See Also: http://www.aha.org/resource/hSTAR.html

Index Medicus (includes *Bibliography of Medical Reviews*). Bethesda, MD, National Library of Medicine, 1960- , monthly, with annual cumulations. Published as author and subject indexes to more than 3,000 journals in the biomedical sciences. Subject headings are based on the controlled vocabulary or thesaurus, *Medical Subject Headings (MeSH).* Since 1966 it has been produced from the MEDLARS database, which provides more comprehensive retrieval, including keyword access and English-language abstracts, than its printed counterparts:

Index Medicus, *International Nursing Index*, and *Index to Dental Literature*.

>   See: *MeSH* terms, such as alcohol drinking; alcoholism; alcoholic intoxication; caffeine; comorbidity; depression; metabolic detoxification, drug; naltrexone; nicotine; smoking; smoking cessation; substance abuse; substance abuse treatment centers; substance dependence; substance withdrawal syndrome; tobacco; tobacco use disorder.

>   See Also: http://www4.ncbi.nlm.nih.gov/PubMed

Index to Scientific Reviews. Philadelphia, Institute for Scientific Information, 1974- , semiannual.

>   See: Permuterm keyword subject index.

>   See: Citation index.

*International Pharmaceutical Abstracts. Washington, DC, American Society of Health-System Pharmacists, 1964- , semimonthly. A key to the world's literature of pharmacy.

>   See: IPA subject terms, such as alcoholism; controlled substances; dependence; drug abuse; drug withdrawal; pharmacotherapy; smoking.

>   See: Subject sections: legislation, laws and regulations; sociology, economics and ethics; toxicology.

*Psychological Abstracts. Washington, DC, American Psychological Association, 1927- , monthly. A compilation of nonevaluative summaries of the world's literature in psychology and related disciplines.

>   See: Index terms, such as addiction; alcohol abuse; alcoholism; alcohol rehabilitation; caffeine; comorbidity; depression; drug abuse; drug addiction; drug dependency; drug rehabilitation; drug therapy; drug usage; drug usage screening; drug withdrawal; naltrexone; nicotine; nicotine withdrawal; social issues; smoking cessation; psychopharmacology; tobacco smoking; treatment outcomes.

>   See Also: http://www.apa.org/psychnet

Public Affairs Information Service Bulletin. New York, Public Affairs Information Service, v.55, 1969- , semimonthly. An index to library material in the field of public affairs and public policy published throughout the world.

> See: PAIS subject headings, such as alcoholism; drug abuse; drug addicts; drugs; smoking.

> See Also: http://www.pais.inter.net

Science Citation Index. Philadelphia, Institute for Scientific Information, 1961- , bimonthly.

> See: Permuterm keyword subject index.

> See: Citation index.

> See Also: http://www.isinet.com

Social Work Abstracts. New York, National Association of Social Workers, v.13, 1977- , quarterly.

> See: Subject index.

Sociological Abstracts. San Diego, CA, Sociological Abstracts, Inc., 1952- , 6 times per year. A collection of nonevaluative abstracts which reflect the world's serial literature in sociology and related disciplines.

> See: *Thesaurus of Sociological Indexing Terms.*

> See: Descriptors such as addict/addicts/addicted/addictive/addiction; alcohol abuse; alcoholism; depression; detoxification; drinking behavior; drug abuse; drug addiction; drug use; habits; smoking; substance abuse; tobacco.

> See Also: http://www.accessinn.com/socabs/index.html

2. CURRENT AWARENESS PUBLICATIONS

Current Contents: Clinical Medicine. Philadelphia, Institute for Scientific Information, v.15, 1987- , weekly.

> See: Keyword index.

Current Contents: Life Sciences. Philadelphia, Institute for Scientific Information, v.10, 1967- , weekly.

See: Keyword index.

Current Contents: Social & Behavioral Sciences. Philadelphia, Institute for Scientific Information, v.6, 1974- , weekly.

See: Keyword index.

3. BOOKS

Medical and Health Care Books and Serials in Print: An Index to Literature in the Health Sciences. New York, R. R. Bowker Co., annual.

See: Library of Congress subject headings, such as alcoholism; drug abuse; drugs; hospitals-outpatient services; narcotic habit; pharmacology; smoking; substance abuse; tobacco.

National Library of Medicine Current Catalog. Bethesda, MD, National Library of Medicine, 1966- , quarterly, with annual cumulations.

See: *MeSH* terms as noted in Section 1 under *Index Medicus.*

Bellenir, Karen. *Substance Abuse Sourcebook.* Detroit, Omnigraphics, 1996.

O'Brien, Robert [and others]. *The Encyclopedia of Drug Abuse.* 2nd ed. New York, Facts on File, c1992.

Stimmel, Barry [and others]. *The Facts About Drug Use: Coping with Drug Use in Your Family, at Work, in Your Community.* Mount Vernon, N.Y., Consumers Union, c1991.

Substance Abuse: The Nation's Number One Health Problem, Key Indicators for Policy. Princeton, NJ, Robert Wood Johnson Foundation, 1993.

Kinney, Jean. *Clinical Manual of Substance Abuse.* St. Louis, Mosby, 1996.

World Health Organization Catalogue: New Books. Geneva, World Health Organization, semiannual (supplements *World Health Organization Publications* and includes periodicals).

See Also: http://www.who.org

4. U.S. GOVERNMENT PUBLICATIONS

Alcohol and Other Drug Thesaurus: A Guide to Concepts and Terminology in Substance Abuse and Addiction (AOD Thesaurus). Rockville, MD, National Institute on Alcohol Abuse and Alcoholism, 2nd ed., 1995.

> See: Title keyword index.

> See Also: http://www.niaaa.nih.gov/publications/thes.htm

*Monthly Catalog of United States Government Publications. Washington, DC, U.S. Government Printing Office, 1895- , monthly.

> See: Keyword index.

> See Also: http://www.access.gpo.gov

5. ONLINE BIBLIOGRAHIC DATABASES

Only those databases which have no print counterparts are included in this section. Print sources which have online database equivalents are noted throughout this guide by the asterisk (*) which appears before the title. If you do not have direct access to these databases, consult your librarian for assistance.

ALCOHOL AND ALCOHOL PROBLEMS SCIENCE DATABASE: ETOH (National Institute on Alcohol Abuse and Alcoholism, Rockville, MD).

> Use: Keywords.

> See Also: http://etoh.niaaa.nih.gov

ALCOHOL INFORMATION FOR CLINICIANS AND EDUCATORS (Project Cork Institute, Dartmouth Medical School, Hanover, NH).

> Use: Keywords.

> See Also: http://www.dartmouth.edu/dms/cork

AMERICAN STATISTICS INDEX (ASI) (Congressional Information Services, Inc., Washington, DC).

   Use: Keywords.

DRUG INFORMATION FULLTEXT (American Society of Health-System Pharmacists, Bethesda, MD).

   Use: Keywords.

DRUGINFO AND ALCOHOL USE AND ABUSE (Hazelden Foundation, Center City, Minn., and Drug Information Service Center, College of Pharmacy, University of Minnesota, Minneapolis, Minn.).

   Use: Keywords.

   See Also: http://www.hazelden.org

LEXIS (LEXIS - NEXIS, Dayton, OH).

   Use: Guide library.

   See Also: http://www.lexis-nexis.com

MAGAZINE DATABASE (Information Access Co., Foster City, CA).

   Use: Keywords.

   See Also: http://www.informationaccess.com/prods/products.html
             http://www.iacnet.com

MENTAL HEALTH ABSTRACTS (MHA) (IFI/Plenum Data Co., Wilmington, NC).

   Use: Keywords.

NATIONAL NEWSPAPER INDEX (Information Access Co., Foster City, CA).

   Use: Keywords.

NTIS (Bibliographic Data Base, U.S. National Technical Information Service, Springfield, VA).

   Use: Keywords.

   See Also: http://www.ntis.gov

PSYCINFO (American Psychological Association, Washington, DC).

> Use: Keywords.

> See Also: http://www.apa.org/psychnet

WESTLAW (West Publishing Co., Eagan, MN).

> Use: Keywords.

> See Also: http://www.westgroup.com

6. HANDBOOKS, DIRECTORIES, GRANT SOURCES, ETC.

Annual Register of Grant Support. Wilmette, Ill., National Register Pub. Co., annual.

> See: Internal medicine; medicine; pharmacology, psychiatry, psychology, mental health sections.

> See: Subject index.

*Biomedical Index to PHS-Supported Research. Bethesda, MD, National Institutes of Health, Division of Research Grants, annual.

> See: Subject index.

Directory of Research Grants. Phoenix, AR, Oryx Press, annual.

> See: Subject index terms, such as alcohol/alcoholism, education, drugs/drug abuse, health promotion.

*Encyclopedia of Associations. Detroit, Gale Research Co., annual (occasional supplements between editions).

> See: Subject index.

*Foundation Directory. New York, The Foundation Center, biennial (updated between editions by *Foundation Directory Supplement*).

> See: Index of foundations.

> See: Index of foundations by state and city.

> See: Index of donors, trustees, and administrators.

> See: Index of fields of interest.

> See Also: http://www.fdncenter.org

Health Hotlines: Toll-Free Numbers from DIRLINE. Bethesda, MD, National Library of Medicine, biennial.

Information Industry Directory. Detroit, Gale Research Co., annual.

Nolan, Kathleen Lopez. *Gale Directory of Databases*. Detroit, Gale Research, Inc., 1996.

Roper, Fred W. and Jo Anne Boorkman. *Introduction to Reference Sources in the Health Sciences*. 3rd ed. Chicago, Medical Library Association, c1994.

The SALIS Directory: Substance Abuse Librarians and Information Specialists. 2nd ed. Berkeley, CA, Alcohol Research Group, Medical Research Institute of San Francisco and University of California, Berkeley, 1991.

Statistics Sources. 21st ed. Detroit, Gale Research Inc., 1997.

7. JOURNAL LISTINGS

The Serials Directory. An International Reference Book. Birmingham, Ebsco Publishing, annual (supplemented by quarterly updates).

Ulrich's International Periodicals Directory, Now Including Irregular Serials & Annuals. New York, R. R. Bowker Co., annual (updated between editions by *Ulrich's Quarterly*).

>   See: Subject categories, such as drug abuse and alcoholism, medical sciences, pharmacy and pharmacology, psychology, public health and safety.

8. AUDIOVISUAL PROGRAMS

The Directory of Medical Video Programs. Hawthorne, NJ, Ridge Publishing Co., 1990.

National Library of Medicine Audiovisuals Catalog. Bethesda, MD, National Library of Medicine, 1977-1993, quarterly, with annual cumulations.

>   See: *MeSH* terms as noted in Section 1 under *Index Medicus*.

Patient Education Sourcebook. 2v. Saint Louis, MO, Health Sciences Communications Association, c1985-90.

  See: *MeSH* terms as noted in Section 1 under *Index Medicus.*

9. GUIDES TO UPCOMING MEETINGS

Scientific Meetings. San Diego, CA, Scientific Meetings Publications, quarterly.

  See: Subject indexes.

  See: Association listing.

World Meetings: Medicine. New York, Macmillan Pub. Co., quarterly.

  See: Keyword index.

  See: Sponsor directory and index.

World Meetings: Social and Behavioral Sciences, Human Services and Management. New York, Macmillan Pub. Co., quarterly.

  See: Keyword index.

  See: Sponsor directory and index.

10. PROCEEDINGS OF MEETINGS

*Directory of Published Proceedings. Series SEMT. Science/Engineering/ Medicine/Technology. Harrison, NY, InterDok Corp., v.3, 1967- , monthly, except July-August, with annual cumulations.

*Index to Scientific and Technical Proceedings. Philadelphia, Institute for Scientific Information, 1978- , monthly with semiannual cumulations.

11. SPECIALIZED RESEARCH CENTERS

Medical Research Centres. Harlow, Essex, Longman, biennial.

International Research Centers Directory. Detroit, Gale Research Co., annual.

Research Centers Directory. Detroit, Gale Research Co., annual (updated by *New Research Centers*).

12. SPECIAL LIBRARY COLLECTIONS

Directory of Special Libraries and Information Centers. Detroit, Gale Research Co., annual (updated by *New Special Libraries*).

Index

In this index, *italic* page numbers designate figures; page numbers followed by "t" designate tables.

Abstinence
  nicotine as assisting in, 4. *See also* Smoking cessation; Withdrawal
  reporting of, 40
  survival effect of, 59-61
Abstracting services, 111-114
Acamprosate, 17
Acting out, 102
Addiction
  compulsive versus repetitive use, 10
  defined, 8-9
  punishment as ineffective in, 10
Addressing Tobacco in the Treatment of Other Addictions Project, 104
Admission criteria, 88-89
Adolescence, as age of onset, 8-9
Adolescents, 2,3
  epidemiologic trends, 18
  smoking prevalence and, 74
African-Americans, 73t,74,88
Age
  alcohol prevalence and, 74
  at onset, 8-9
  smoking prevalence and, 74
  survival rate and, 61
Aggressive behavior, 99
Alcoholics, resistance to nicotine detoxification, 12
Alcoholics Anonymous (AA), survival study, 59-60

Alcoholism, 3,55-66. *See also* Alcohol use
  abstinence as related to mortality, 59-61
  comorbidity with smoking, 16,61-62
  epidemiology, 56t,56-57
  morbidity, 59
  mortality, 57-58,62
  predictors of mortality, 58
  smokefree environment study, 83-108. *See also* Smokefree program
  smoking as marker for, 15
  societal costs, 58
  success rates for treatment, 13
Alcohol use. *See also* Alcoholism
  epidemiology, 68-69
  prevalence in primary care population, 74-77,75t,76t. *See also* Primary care study
Alina Lodge (New Jersey) cessation study, 84
Anhedonia, 8,11. *See also* Depression; Withdrawal
Antidepressants, 15,42,44-45. *See also* Depression
Anxiety, 49,99
Asian-American study populations, 73t,74
Attitudes, of staff, 100-101,103-104
Attrition, 87-88,91,93t-97t

Beck Depression Inventory, 38,43,48
Behavior, 99
Behavior therapy, 44-45
Beta-endorphins, 10,17
Bibliographical databases, 116-118
Biological basis of addiction, 2,7-11
    addiction/dependence patterns, 8-9
    in brain, 7-11
    genetic factors, 9
    long-term brain effects, 10-11
    monoamine oxidase B (MAO B)
        inhibition, 23-34
    neurobiology, 9-10
Brain glucose metabolism, 27-31,*30*.
    See also Monoamine
        oxidase B (MAO B)
        inhibition
Brain patterns of addiction, 9-10
Buproprion, 44

Caffeine, 3
    inpatient comorbidity study of,
        47-54
    literature review, 48-50
    sources of, 51
CAGE screening, 70,78
Cancer, 62,69
Caregivers, smoking by, 100-101
Center for Epidemiologic Studies
        Depression Scale (CES-D),
        42
Clonidine therapy, 17
Clonidine trials, of depression and
        smoking cessation, 36-45.
        See also Depression
Cocaine, 2,10,11. *See also* Drug
        dependency
Comorbidity. *See also* Depression
    alcohol addiction, 55-66. *See also*
        Alcoholism
    alcohol use, 49
    drug dependence, 16,47-54
    mortality and, 62

psychiatric, 15-16,35-46,44,
        47-54,52t,62
    significance of nicotine addiction
        treatment in, 104-105
Compulsive drug seeking, 15
Compulsive versus repetitive use, 10
Cost effectiveness, 13-14
Counseling, 44-45
CPC Packwood Hospital (Atlanta,
        GA) cessation study, 85

Death certificate studies, 61-62
L-Deprenyl in Parkinson's disease,
        2,24
Depression, 3,15,35-46
    clinical implications of study, 43
    depressed mood during nicotine
        withdrawal, 37,*38*
    gender factors in, 37,42
    recurrence rate of, 42
    research implications of study,
        44-45
    severe after smoking cessation,
        37-43,39t,*40*,41t
Detoxification, 18,90. *See also*
    Withdrawal
    addict preferences in, 12
Developmental theories of addiction,
        10
Dopaminergic pathways, 2,9-11,12
Doxepin, 44
Drug dependence, 3. *See also*
        Comorbidity
    concurrent caffeine and nicotine
        use in, 47-54
    epidemiology, 68-69
    prevalence, 77
    in primary care population, 67-81.
        See also Primary care study
    smoke-free environment in
        treatment, 83-108
    success rates for treatment, 13
DSM-IIIR criteria, 88
DSM-IV criteria, 11,48,88

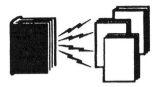

Haworth
DOCUMENT DELIVERY
SERVICE

This valuable service provides a single-article order form for any article from a Haworth journal.

- *Time Saving:* No running around from library to library to find a specific article.
- *Cost Effective:* All costs are kept down to a minimum.
- *Fast Delivery:* Choose from several options, including same-day FAX.
- *No Copyright Hassles:* You will be supplied by the original publisher.
- *Easy Payment:* Choose from several easy payment methods.

Open Accounts Welcome for ...
- Library Interlibrary Loan Departments
- Library Network/Consortia Wishing to Provide Single-Article Services
- Indexing/Abstracting Services with Single Article Provision Services
- Document Provision Brokers and Freelance Information Service Providers

---

MAIL or *FAX* THIS ENTIRE ORDER FORM TO:

Haworth Document Delivery Service
The Haworth Press, Inc.
10 Alice Street
Binghamton, NY 13904-1580

or FAX: 1-800-895-0582
or CALL: 1-800-342-9678
9am-5pm EST

PLEASE SEND ME PHOTOCOPIES OF THE FOLLOWING SINGLE ARTICLES:

1) Journal Title: _____
   Vol/Issue/Year: _____ Starting & Ending Pages: _____
   Article Title: _____
   _____

2) Journal Title: _____
   Vol/Issue/Year: _____ Starting & Ending Pages: _____
   Article Title: _____
   _____

3) Journal Title: _____
   Vol/Issue/Year: _____ Starting & Ending Pages: _____
   Article Title: _____
   _____

4) Journal Title: _____
   Vol/Issue/Year: _____ Starting & Ending Pages: _____
   Article Title: _____
   _____

(See other side for Costs and Payment Information)

COSTS: Please figure your cost to order quality copies of an article.

1. Set-up charge per article: $8.00
   ($8.00 × number of separate articles) _____

2. Photocopying charge for each article:

   1-10 pages: $1.00 _____

   11-19 pages: $3.00 _____

   20-29 pages: $5.00 _____

   30+ pages: $2.00/10 pages _____

3. Flexicover (optional): $2.00/article _____

4. Postage & Handling: US: $1.00 for the first article/

   $.50 each additional article _____

   Federal Express: $25.00 _____

   Outside US: $2.00 for first article/
   $.50 each additional article_____

5. Same-day FAX service: $.35 per page _____

                                GRAND TOTAL: _____

METHOD OF PAYMENT: (please check one)

❑ Check enclosed   ❑ Please ship and bill. PO # _____
                   (sorry we can ship and bill to bookstores only! All others must pre-pay)

❑ Charge to my credit card: ❑ Visa; ❑ MasterCard; ❑ Discover;
                             ❑ American Express;

Account Number:_____ Expiration date:_____

Signature: ✗_____

Name: _____ Institution: _____

Address: _____

_____

City: _____ State:_____ Zip:_____

Phone Number: _____ FAX Number: _____

MAIL or *FAX* THIS ENTIRE ORDER FORM TO:

Haworth Document Delivery Service	**or FAX:** 1-800-895-0582
The Haworth Press, Inc.	**or CALL:** 1-800-342-9678
10 Alice Street	9am-5pm EST)
Binghamton, NY 13904-1580	